Workbook for the Identification of Phonological Processes and Distinctive Features

FOURTH EDITION

Robert J. Lowe

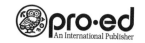

pro·ed
An International Publisher

8700 Shoal Creek Boulevard
Austin, TX 78757
800-897-3202   Fax: 800-397-7633
www.proedinc.com

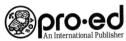

© 1989, 1996, 2002, 2010 by PRO-ED, Inc.
8700 Shoal Creek Boulevard
Austin, Texas 78757-6897
800/897-3202   Fax 800/397-7633
www.proedinc.com

ISBN: 978-1-4164-0437-8

Art Director: Jason Crosier
Designer: Lissa Hattersley
This book is designed in Minion and Neutra Text.

Printed in the United States of America

1 2 3 4 5 6 7 8 9 10   18 17 16 15 14 13 12 11 10 09

Workbook for the Identification of Phonological Processes and Distinctive Features

This workbook is dedicated to my wife of 32 years.
Thank you, Bonnie, for your unwavering support and continued love.
All of my love, always.

CONTENTS ◇◇◇◇◇◇◇◇◇◇◇◇◇◇◇◇◇◇◇◇◇◇◇◇◇◇◇◇◇◇◇◇◇◇◇◇◇

◇◇◇

EXERCISE 8 ◇◇

DIRECTIONS: To recognize phonological processes, the clinician must be able to identify phonetic contexts in which processes are likely to occur. For each of the following target words, place a check mark in the column(s) of the process(es) that could occur. In the example, across from the target word *boat* there are check marks for final- and initial-consonant deletion. The other processes (syllable deletion, reduplication, epenthesis, cluster deletion, and cluster substitution) are not likely to occur in one-syllable words without clusters.

Target Word	Syllable Deletion	Reduplication	Epenthesis	Final-Consonant Deletion	Initial-Consonant Deletion	Cluster Deletion	Cluster Substitution
Ex: *boat*				✓	✓		
1. bed				✓	✓		
2. goat				✓	✓		
3. grape			✓	✓		✓	✓
4. bucket	✓			✓	✓		
5. nest			✓		✓	✓	✓
6. mouse				✓	✓		
7. tribe			✓	✓	✓	✓	✓
8. cry			✓			✓	✓
9. stone			✓	✓		✓	✓
10. ouch				✓			
11. tomato	✓	✓			✓		
12. tan				✓	✓		
13. east			✓			✓	✓
14. stray			✓			✓	✓
15. trapper	✓	✓	✓			✓	✓

EXERCISE 9

DIRECTIONS: Show the effects of initial- and final-consonant deletion and cluster reduction for the following words. For each word with a cluster, there will be three possibilities for cluster deletion.

Target	Initial-Consonant Deletion	Final-Consonant Deletion	Cluster Deletion
Ex: *stoop*	NA	[stu]	[tup] or [sup] or [up]
1. taste	_____	_____	_____
2. seed	_____	_____	_____
3. steep	_____	_____	_____
4. slip	_____	_____	_____
5. bread	_____	_____	_____
6. road	_____	_____	_____
7. park	_____	_____	_____
8. plate	_____	_____	_____
9. mash	_____	_____	_____
10. brave	_____	_____	_____

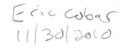

EXERCISE 14 ⬦⬦⬦⬦⬦⬦⬦⬦⬦⬦⬦⬦⬦⬦⬦⬦⬦⬦⬦⬦⬦⬦⬦⬦⬦

DIRECTIONS: For each word listed below, determine what sound changes have occurred and place a check mark in the appropriate process column(s).

Target	Child Form	Sound Change	Syllable Deletion	Reduplication	Epenthesis	Final-Consonant Deletion	Initial-Consonant Deletion	Cluster Deletion	Cluster Substitution
Ex: *boat*	[bo]	t → Ø				✓			
1. bed	[ɛd]	b → Ø					✓		
2. goat	[o]	g → Ø t → Ø				✓	✓		
3. grape	[gəreɪ]	gr → gər			✓	✓			
4. bucket	[bʌbɑ]	CVCVC → CVCV	✓			✓			
5. nest	[nɛt]	st → t						✓	
6. mouse	[maʊ]	s → Ø				✓			
7. tribe	[twaɪ]	tr → tw · b → Ø				✓			✓
8. cry	[kaɪ]	kr → k						✓	
9. stone	[on]	st → Ø						✓	
10. ouch	[aʊ]	tʃ → Ø				✓			
11. tomato	[meɪdo]	CVCVCV → CVCV	✓				✓	✓	✓
12. tan	[æn]	t → Ø					✓		
13. east	[it]	st → t						✓	
14. stray	[tweɪ]	str → tw						✓	✓
15. trapper	[təræpə]	tr → tər ər → ə			✓				

⬦⬦⬦⬦⬦⬦⬦⬦⬦⬦⬦⬦⬦⬦⬦⬦⬦⬦⬦⬦⬦⬦⬦⬦⬦⬦⬦⬦⬦⬦⬦⬦⬦⬦⬦⬦⬦⬦

EXERCISE 12 ◇◇◇

DIRECTIONS: For each of the following examples, distinguish between total and partial reduplication.

Target	Child Form	Answer
1. water	[wɑwɑ]	_____
2. blanket	[didi]	_____
3. bottle	[bɑdɑ]	_____
4. daddy	[dædɑ]	_____
5. candy	[kɑki]	_____
6. pillow	[pɑpo]	_____
7. puppy	[pɑpɑ]	_____
8. nanny	[nɑnɑ]	_____
9. bottle	[bɑbi]	_____
10. baby	[beɪbe]	_____

EXERCISE 13 ◇◇◇

DIRECTIONS: Show the effects of epenthesis on each of the following words.

Target	Answer
1. space	_____
2. train	_____
3. play	_____
4. black	_____
5. steak	_____

◇◇

ACKNOWLEDGMENTS

The author gratefully acknowledges the aid of his past teaching assistants during the development and subsequent revisions of this workbook. In particular, Marlo Yenser, Eliza Newcomer, and Meghan Allshouse are commended for their work on the project. I would also like to thank Beth Donnelly, Senior Editor with PRO-ED, Inc., who encouraged and supported the most recent revisions.

PREFACE

The field of speech–language pathology continues to employ the use of phonological processes or patterns as a means to summarize and describe error patterns found in the speech of children. The field also continues to use distinctive features in developing theories and in exploring new means of examining speech errors. This workbook provides basic information describing both processes and distinctive features along with practice items to facilitate application of the material. New to this fourth edition are some needed corrections to the last edition and added content related to revisions of phonology tests and new assessment instruments.

INTRODUCTION

The field of speech–language pathology has witnessed a remarkable growth in the area of phonology over the past decade. *Phonology,* a term once restricted to linguistics, has become commonplace in speech–language pathology. Along with phonology comes the term *phonological process.* Stampe (1973) introduced the concept of phonological processes to explain systematic sound changes made by children in producing adult words. As children grow, these processes are suppressed or eliminated until the child's phonological system matches that of the adults. Speech–language pathologists now use the term *phonological processes* to describe sound-change patterns that occur in children's speech.

This workbook is about phonology and phonological processes. It is intended to provide background and practice for clinicians and students who will be assessing children with phonological disabilities.

In recent years, the term *phonological process* has been associated with the literature on reading development. In that context, it refers to the ability to use phonological information in processing written and oral language. In referring to sound change errors, Hodson and others have encouraged a change to the term *phonological pattern* rather than *process* to avoid confusion. However, the original label, *phonological process,* continues to be used by the field in textbooks, assessment instruments, and journal articles. For this workbook, the terms *process* and *pattern* will be used interchangeably, with a preference for the term *process.*

Articulation and Phonology

One change brought about by the increased interest in phonology has been in the use of the terms *articulation* and *phonology.* While some writers use the two terms interchangeably, the current trend is to make a distinction between them.

Phonology is a broader term that refers to the organization and classification of speech sounds that occur as contrastive units within a given language (Stoel-Gammon & Dunn, 1985). A simpler definition was supplied by Edwards and Shriberg (1983), who defined phonology as the study of the sound component of language.

Both definitions refer to phonology as part of the language system. Ingram (1982) described this shift as a general trend in the research, which has moved from a study of how a child produces sounds to a study of sound production in the context of the linguistic system. In his words, "The phonologist is not just concerned with whether or not 'f' is produced, but also with target sounds and the contrastive status of substitutions" (p. 1).

Articulation has come to be viewed as one part of phonology. It is referred to as the overt level of speech production, which consists of the speech sounds we hear and produce (Edwards & Shriberg, 1983). Articulation relates to the physical movements and motor abilities that are required to produce speech sounds.

Phonology also has a *covert* level, or level of phonological knowledge. Edwards and Shriberg (1983) designated four parts to this level: (a) an inventory of contrastive sounds (phonemes), (b) morpheme structure rules and sequential constraints that determine permissible word and syllable formations, (c) morphophonemic rules for correctly producing combinations of morphemes, and (d) allophonic rules for correctly producing allophones of phonemes.

Phonology is one of five components of the language system, the others being syntax, semantics, morphology, and pragmatics. Edwards and Shriberg (1983) described the relationship between these components and phonology: "These other components and functions are concerned with choice and ordering of words in accordance with appropriate social contexts and individual histories, needs, and intentions. The task of the phonological component is to translate the message into manifest speech" (p. 37).

Phonological Processes

A comparison of adult and child phonological systems reveals that child speech production errors are typically simplifications of adult models. These simplifications are not random. For example, a child does not substitute a [w] for /r/ during one production and a [t] for /r/ the next. Instead, the substitutions are fairly consistent. Some variation is expected due to phonetic context and the fact that the child is in the process of learning the adult system, but generally once the system is known, errors are predictable. In fact, once the adult figures out the system, the child's intelligibility greatly increases.

Children with more severe articulation problems also demonstrate predictable errors. These children show systematic patterns of sound change that affect whole classes of sounds. These sound-change patterns are referred to as *phonological processes* or *patterns,* and they can influence classes of sounds or sound sequences. For example, one common phonological process is *stopping,* in which fricative sounds are replaced by stop-plosives.

DEFINITION ——————————————————————————————

A phonological process is a systematic sound change that affects classes of sounds or sound sequences and results in a simplification of production.

It should be noted that the sound change does not have to affect all the sounds within a class, but it must affect at least two. In the example of stopping, there are nine fricatives that might be affected. If only two of them were systematically changed to stops, this could still be labeled stopping, because two is the smallest sampling that can still be considered a class of sounds. Simply put, one sound error in a class does not make a process.

Other criteria for identifying phonological processes have been suggested. McReynolds and Elbert (1981), for example, demonstrated how criteria could significantly change identification results. In their study they suggested that a sound change should have the possibility of occurring four times and be used at least 20% of the time before qualifying as a process. At present no standardized criteria have been established for the identification of processes. On most of the published phonology instruments, if a particular sound change occurs even once, it identifies a phonological process.

It is suggested that in identifying processes the clinician keep the following in mind as minimal requirements for qualifying a sound change as a phonological process:

1. A process must affect more than one sound from a given sound class.
2. The sound change must occur at least 40% of the time.

Processes Affecting Consonants

Several phonological processes have been identified in the research literature. As early as 1980, Shriberg and Kwiatkowski listed more than 40 processes in their text on natural process analysis. Ingram (1989) suggested grouping these processes into three categories: (a) processes that affect the syllable shape of words, (b) processes that substitute one sound for another, and (c) processes that result in sounds becoming more like other sounds (assimilation). Bernthal and Bankson (1993) suggested two categories: (a) whole-word processes, which simplify a word or syllable structure and segmental contrast within a word, and (b) segment change processes, which involve some form of substitution for specific segments or types of segments, regardless of syllable or word position. Since Ingram's system has been used more frequently, the processes covered by this book and presented in Table 1 are grouped by syllable structure, substitution, and assimilation processes.

TABLE 1

Phonological Processes Involving Consonants and/or Syllables

Syllable Structure Processes	Substitution Processes	Assimilation Processes
Syllable deletion	Stopping	Labial assimilation
Reduplication	Stridency deletion	Alveolar assimilation
Epenthesis	Fronting	Velar assimilation
Final consonant deletion	Depalatalization	Nasal assimilation
Initial consonant deletion	Palatalization	Prevocalic voicing
Cluster deletion	Affrication	Postvocalic devoicing
Cluster substitution	Deaffrication	Metathesis
	Backing	Coalescence
	Alveolarization	

Processes Affecting Vowels

In addition to discussing processes affecting consonants, this workbook presents information and exercises dealing with vowel processes. Vowel processes are sound changes that affect vowels.

DEFINITION ————————————————————————————————

A vowel process is a systematic vowel change that affects features, complexity, or vowel harmony.

Feature changes are changes in vowel height, frontness, or roundness. Complexity changes occur when the vowel quality changes from monophthong to diphthong or from diphthong to monophthong. Vowel harmony changes occur when a vowel change is influenced by phonetic context. The vowel processes discussed in this workbook are presented in Table 2.

Workbook Format

The format of this workbook is simple. Groups of phonological processes are presented along with their definitions. The definitions may vary according to different phonology assessment instruments, and any such variations are pointed out. Exercises are provided at the end of each major section to help the reader develop a working knowledge of various processes, in many cases following formats used by the most common phonology assessment instruments. Answers to these exercises, and to two mini-quizzes, appear at the end of the book.

Phonological processes from the following instruments were used in developing this workbook (abbreviations are used throughout):

ALPHA Test of Phonology–Revised
   (ALPHA–R; Lowe, 2000)

Bankson–Bernthal Test of Phonology
   (BBTOP; Bankson & Bernthal, 1990)

TABLE 2
Phonological Processes Involving Vowel Changes

Feature Change Processes	Complexity Changes	Vowel Harmony Processes
Vowel backing	Diphthongization	Tenseness harmony
Vowel lowering	Diphthong reduction	Height harmony
Vowel raising		Complete vowel harmony
Centralization		
Vowel unrounding		

Clinical Assessment of Articulation and Phonology
  (CAAP; Secord & Donohue, 2002)

Diagnostic Evaluation of Articulation and Phonology
  (DEAP; Dodd, Hua, Crosbie, Holm, & Ozanne, 2006)

Hodson Assessment of Phonological Patterns–Third Edition
  (HAPP-3; Hodson, 2004)

Khan-Lewis Phonological Analysis–Second Edition
  (KLPA-2; Khan & Lewis, 2002)

Smit–Hand Articulation and Phonology Evaluation
  (SHAPE; Smit & Hand, 1997)

Structured Photographic Articulation Test featuring Dudberry II
  (SPAT-D II; Dawson & Tattersall, 2001)

These tests are described in the Appendix.

CHAPTER 1

Consonant and Vowel Review

The recognition of phonological processes often involves the identification of changes in place, manner, and/or voicing features of speech sounds. For example, the process of stopping can be identified by recognizing that stop-plosives systematically replace fricatives. Place, manner, and voicing are also involved in determining production deficits (e.g., class deficiencies on the HAPP-3) and summarizing production constraints (e.g., ALPHA–R).

Recent assessment practices have described systematic changes in vowels as vowel processes. As with consonants, the identification of vowel processes requires a thorough understanding of the basic tongue height, advancement, and rounding features used in distinguishing the various English vowels.

This section provides a thorough review of cosonant and vowel features. It is recommended that the reader understand this section very well before moving on to the process definitions and exercises. Time spent at this point is crucial for developing a firm foundation in working with and understanding phonological processes.

Place, Manner, and Voicing

Any English consonant can be identified if its place, manner, and voicing characteristics are known. *Place* refers to the point in the vocal tract where the sound is made; *manner* refers to the way in which the sound is produced; and *voice* refers to the presence or absence of vocal-fold vibration during the production of the speech sound. Table 3 shows a breakdown of English consonants based on their place, manner, and voicing features.

Place

Place indicates where a speech sound is formed. More specifically, place is determined by the point in the vocal tract where most closure or constriction occurs in the production of the

TABLE 3

Place, Manner, and Voicing Characteristics of English Consonants

Place	Plosives VL	Plosives V	Fricatives VL	Fricatives V	Affricates VL	Affricates V	Nasals V	Liquids V	Glides V
Bilabial	p	b					m		w
Labio-dental			f	v					
Lingua-dental			θ	ð					
Lingua-alveolar	t	d	s	z			n	l	
Palatal			ʃ	ʒ	ʧ	ʤ		r	j
Velar	k	g					ŋ		
Glottal	ʔ		h						

speech sound. The places of articulation occur at several points along the vocal tract, beginning at the lips and ending at the glottis. Awareness of place is important to the speech–language pathologist. Some sound changes can be described by the changes in place that occur. For example, the process of *fronting* can be defined as the substitution of a more anterior sound for a velar. Unless the clinician is aware of the place relationships among sounds, identification of this process will be difficult.

Bilabial. Bilabial is the most anterior of the places of articulation. Bilabial means "two lips"; thus, consonants that are produced using both lips fall into this category. The bilabial consonants include /p/, /b/, /m/, and /w/. Some descriptions also include the voiceless "w", which is symbolized as /hw/ or /ʍ/.

Labio-dental. Sounds that are made with both the lips and the central incisors are called labio-dental. These sounds are produced with contact between the lower lip and the bottom edge of the upper incisors. The labio-dental sounds include /f/ and /v/.

> NOTE: The bilabial and labio-dental sounds are referred to together as the labial sounds.

Lingua-dental (interdental). Sounds made with the tongue touching the bottom edge of the upper central incisors or the backs of the central incisors are called lingua-dental or interdental. The two interdental sounds are /θ/ and /ð/.

Lingua-alveolar. Immediately behind the upper central incisors is the alveolar ridge area. Several speech sounds are made with the major constriction in this area. The actual place of articulation on the ridge varies due to the influence of the phonetic context in which the sounds occur. The lingua-alveolar (or simply *alveolar*) sounds include /t/, /d/, /n/, /s/, /z/, and /l/.

Lingua-palatal. The lingua-palatal or *palatal* place of articulation lies just posterior to the alveolar ridge, about where the rugae are located and where the vault angles upward. The palatal sounds include /ʃ/, /ʒ/, /tʃ/, /dʒ/, /r/, and /j/.

> NOTE: The boundary between the palatal area and the alveolar ridge is often used as the landmark between anterior and posterior places of articulation in categorizing distinctive features. This area is sometimes referred to as the palatal-alveolar place of articulation.

Lingua-velar. The lingua-velar or *velar* place of articulation is located at the back of the oral cavity, posterior to the palatal area and just anterior to the uvula. The velar sounds include /k/, /g/, and /ŋ/.

Glottal. The glottis is the opening between the vocal folds. Sounds made at this location are /h/ and the glottal stop /ʔ/. The glottal stop is not one of the standard speech sounds of American English; however, it is included here, as it is a substitution often heard in children's speech.

Manner

Manner refers to the way speech sounds are made. More accurately, it refers to the way the airstream is modified in the production of speech sounds. It can also refer to the degree of closure that is used during the sound production.

Plosives. Plosives are also referred to as *stops* or as *stop-plosives*. They are formed by a complete closure of the vocal tract, including the velopharyngeal port, so that the flow of the outgoing airstream is temporarily stopped. Pressure builds up behind this closure so that when the airstream is released, an "explosion" results. The plosive sounds include /p/, /b/, /t/, /d/, /k/, /g/, and the glottal stop /ʔ/. The phonological process of stopping derives its name from this manner, because it describes a sound change wherein stops systematically replace fricatives.

Fricatives. Fricatives describe speech sounds that are produced by directing the airstream through a narrow constriction in the vocal tract. The forcing of the air through the constriction creates turbulence or friction. There are nine fricatives: /f/, /v/, /θ/, /ð/, /s/, /z/, /ʃ/, /ʒ/, and /h/.

Affricates. An affricate is usually considered to be a combination of a stop and a fricative. The stop component occurs first, followed by the fricative segment. There are two affricates: /tʃ/, and /dʒ/.

> NOTE: Affricates and the noisy fricatives are sometimes grouped together. They form the class of sounds called stridents. The stridents include /f/, /v/, /s/, /z/, /ʃ/, /tʃ/, and /dʒ/. The stridents do not include the /h/, / θ/, or /ð/ sounds.

Nasals. The nasal sounds are produced by making a complete closure along the vocal tract but leaving the velopharyngeal port open. As a result, part of the airstream is directed through the nasal cavity. The three nasal consonants are /m/, /n/, and /ŋ/.

Liquids. Liquids are vowel-like consonants that have only slightly more closure in their production than the vowels do. The closure is not sufficient to result in any friction-like noise. The two liquids are /l/ and /r/.

Glides. Glides, like liquids, are similar to vowels in their production. The glides, however, include a shift in placement from a more closed to a more open position. How far the position is open depends on the vowel that follows the glide. The glides (also called *semivowels*) include /j/ and /w/.

> NOTE: Glides and liquids together are sometimes referred to as *approximants*.

Obstruents. The term *obstruent* refers to sounds that are made with enough constriction of the vocal tract to impede or obstruct the airstream. Obstruents include the combined manners of stops, fricatives, and affricates.

Sonorants. The term *sonorants* is used to describe the grouping of nasals, liquids, and glides. Sonorancy means that the consonant has a vowel-like quality. As noted in their descriptions, the liquids and glides are made with a very open vocal tract, and the nasals have an open velopharyngeal port. The sounds in these classes are also all produced with formants.

Voicing

The voicing characteristics of the English consonants fall into two categories: voiced and voiceless. In general, all of the obstruents have voiced and voiceless pairs called *cognates.* The nasals, liquids, and glides tend to be only voiced.

Work Exercises 1 through 4 to help you develop an understanding of place, manner, and voicing.

EXERCISE 1 ◇◇

DIRECTIONS: Indicate the speech sound that is described by the following characteristics.

Characteristics	Speech Sound
1. Voiced, lingua-alveolar, plosive	_____
2. Voiceless, lingua-dental, fricative	_____
3. Voiced, palatal, glide	_____
4. Voiced, labio-dental, fricative	_____
5. Voiced, velar, nasal	_____
6. Voiced, palatal, fricative	_____
7. Voiceless, lingua-alveolar, plosive	_____
8. Voiceless, palatal, affricate	_____
9. Voiced, lingua-alveolar, liquid	_____
10. Voiced, velar, plosive	_____

EXERCISE 2 ◇◇

DIRECTIONS: Provide the voicing, place, and manner for the following sounds.

Sound	Voicing	Place	Manner
1. /w/	_____	_____	_____
2. /z/	_____	_____	_____
3. /h/	_____	_____	_____
4. /b/	_____	_____	_____
5. /f/	_____	_____	_____
6. /ʃ/	_____	_____	_____
7. /n/	_____	_____	_____
8. /dʒ/	_____	_____	_____
9. /k/	_____	_____	_____
10. /r/	_____	_____	_____

⬥⬥⬥⬥⬥⬥ EXERCISE 3 ⬥⬥⬥⬥⬥⬥⬥⬥⬥⬥⬥⬥⬥⬥⬥⬥⬥⬥⬥⬥⬥⬥⬥⬥⬥⬥⬥⬥

DIRECTIONS: Indicate the sounds that belong in the following groups.

Group	Sounds
1. All voiced labials	_____
2. All voiced fricatives	_____
3. All velars	_____
4. All palatals	_____
5. All nonstrident fricatives	_____
6. All strident lingual fricatives	_____
7. All strident nonfricatives	_____
8. All strident obstruents	_____
9. All voiceless, labial obstruents	_____
10. All palatal fricatives	_____

⬥⬥⬥⬥⬥⬥ EXERCISE 4 ⬥⬥⬥⬥⬥⬥⬥⬥⬥⬥⬥⬥⬥⬥⬥⬥⬥⬥⬥⬥⬥⬥⬥⬥⬥⬥⬥⬥

DIRECTIONS: Tell what the sounds in each group have in common.

Sounds	Group
1. /v/, /b/, /m/	_____
2. /d/, /n/, /s/, /z/	_____
3. /h/, /θ/, /ð/	_____
4. /b/, /g/, /d/	_____
5. /j/, /r/, /ʃ/, /ʧ/, /ʤ/, /ʒ/	_____
6. /ʧ/, /t/, /s/, /k/, /p/	_____
7. /k/, /g/, /ŋ/	_____
8. /z/, /ʒ/, /v/, /ð/	_____
9. /ʃ/, /ʧ/	_____
10. /θ/, /s/, /ʃ/, /f/	_____

Vowel System

Like consonants, the various vowels of American English can be identified based on a few features or characteristics. These characteristics include height, frontness, rounding, and tenseness. Vowels are divided into two groups: monophthongs and diphthongs.

Monophthongs (pure vowels) are vowels that have a single, unchanging vowel quality. In contrast, diphthongs are vowels whose quality changes during their production. Diphthongs are symbolized using two symbols (digraph), whereas most monophthongs are designated using one symbol. In this review we will begin with the pure vowels and then cover the diphthongs.

Pure Vowels (Monophthongs)

The pure vowels constitute most of the vowel system and can be distinguished from one another based on two features: tongue height and tongue advancement. The features of rounding and tenseness can be used to make finer distinctions.

Figure 1 is a vowel quadrangle that roughly shows the tongue height and advancement for producing the various pure vowels. The vertical dimension represents tongue height, and the horizontal dimension represents tongue advancement. Thus the quadrangle indicates that the vowel /i/ is made with a high, front positioning of the tongue.

The pure vowels are typically divided into three series—front, central, and back—based on tongue advancement. That convention will be followed here. As we go through these series, vowel height, rounding, and tenseness will also be discussed. Vowel height is used to distinguish among the vowels in a series. Rounding refers to lip configuration during vowel production. Muscular activity is noted by the terms *tense* and *lax*. Tense vowels are produced with a greater degree of muscular activity and duration than lax vowels are. The distinction can be

Front	Central	Back	
/i/		/u/	High
/ɪ/		/ʊ/	High-mid
/e/	/ɝ/ /ə/ /ɚ/	/o/	Mid
/ɛ/	/ʌ/	/ɔ/	Low-mid
/æ/		/ɑ/	Low

FIGURE 1. Vowel quadrangle.

experienced by producing the /i/ and /ɪ/ vowels. The first is tense, and the second lax. For a more detailed description of the vowels, the reader is referred to Shriberg and Kent's (1995) textbook, *Clinical Phonetics*.

Front Series Vowels. The front series gets its name because in producing these vowels, the tongue is positioned toward the front of the mouth. The series includes the vowels /i/, /ɪ/, /e/, /ɛ/, and /æ/. As noted, tongue height distinguishes the vowels from one another within the series. The vowel made with the highest tongue position is the /i/. This vowel is made with the lips unrounded, and it is considered a tense vowel.

The /ɪ/ is made with a slightly lowered and more central tongue position called high-mid. It is also unrounded but is considered a lax vowel. The mid-front series vowel is the /e/. This vowel has a diphthong version as well, /eɪ/. The /eɪ/ is unrounded and is considered a tense vowel. Made with a slightly lower tongue positioning, the /ɛ/ is the next vowel in the series and occupies the low-mid position. The lips are unrounded in producing this vowel, and it is considered lax.

The final vowel in the front series is the /æ/. It is the lowest of the front vowels. This vowel is usually considered to be tense, because it has a longer duration than its neighbor, the /ɛ/. The /æ/ is made with the lips unrounded.

Central Series Vowels. The vowels of the central series are all made with the tongue body near the center of the mouth. We will consider four vowels in this series: /ɝ/, /ə/, /ɚ/, and /ʌ/. There is little difference in the tongue position for these vowels. As can be seen in Figure 1, the /ʌ/ and /ə/ (called the *schwa*) tend to be made with a lower tongue position, and the /ʌ/ is made with the tongue in the back central area. Of these two, the schwa is produced in unstressed syllables and the /ʌ/ used in stressed syllables. For example, the word *above* would be transcribed [əbʌv] as the second syllable is pronounced with more stress than the first.

Both the /ɚ/ (called the *schwar*) and the /ɝ/ have r-coloring in their production. These two vowels are also rounded, but the degree of rounding will vary with the speaker and can even be absent without significantly affecting vowel quality. The schwar is considered the lax member of the pair. In combination with pure vowels, the schwar forms the various rhotic diphthongs.

Back Series Vowels. The tongue is positioned near the back of the oral cavity for the production of the back series vowels. All of these vowels are produced with lip rounding, with the exception of the /ɑ/. The /u/ is made with the highest tongue position. This vowel is tense and rounded. The vowel made with a slightly lower and more central tongue position is the /ʊ/. This vowel, considered lax, is made with rounded lips and occupies the high-mid position on the quadrangle.

The mid-back series vowel is the /o/, which is tense and also rounded. It has a diphthong counterpart, the /oʊ/. Below this is found the /ɔ/, a tense, rounded vowel in the low-mid position. The vowel made with the lowest tongue position is the /ɑ/. This is the only back vowel that is not rounded. Some texts consider this vowel to be tense, and others list it as lax.

Work Exercises 5 and 6, which cover knowledge of monophthongs.

EXERCISE 5 ◇◇

DIRECTIONS: Indicate the vowel associated with the following features.

Features	Vowel
1. High-mid, front	_____
2. Low-mid, back	_____
3. Mid, front	_____
4. Low-mid, front	_____
5. Low-mid, central	_____
6. High-mid, back	_____
7. Low, back	_____
8. Mid-central, tense, rounded	_____
9. Mid-back	_____
10. Low, front	_____

EXERCISE 6 ◇◇

DIRECTIONS: Below is a blank vowel quadrangle. Fill in the missing vowels.

	Front	Central	Back	
	/ /		/ /	High
	/ /		/ /	High-mid
	/ /	/ / / / / /	/ /	Mid
	/ /	/ /	/ /	Low-mid
	/ /		/ /	Low

Diphthongs

Diphthongs are vowels produced with a gradually changing vowel quality. They have two components, an onglide and an offglide. The onglide is the vowel the diphthong begins with, and the offglide is the vowel to which it changes. Typically, the offglide has a higher tongue position than the onglide. Because two vowels are involved in their production, diphthongs are symbolized with digraphs. Some systems include a bar line above or below the digraph (e.g., /a͟ʊ/ or /a͞ʊ/) to indicate that the two sounds function together. This line is called a *ligature*.

American English diphthongs are of two types: phonemic and nonphonemic. Phonemic diphthongs are those that cannot be reduced to monophthongs without affecting the meaning of the words in which they are found. There are three phonemic diphthongs: /ɑɪ/, /ɔɪ/, and /ɑʊ/, as used in the words *bye, toy,* and *cow,* respectively.

The nonphonemic diphthongs were noted in the discussion of pure vowels as counterparts to the /e/ and /o/ monophthongs. They are /eɪ/ and /oʊ/. These two diphthongs can be reduced to monophthongs without changing word meaning. Thus *rope* could be produced with either the diphthong or the monophthong and be recognized as the same word. The diphthong versions of these two sounds usually occur in stressed syllables, while the monophthong versions occur in weakly stressed syllables.

Rhotic Diphthongs. Diphthongs formed with the schwar vowel make up the rhotic diphthongs. They are symbolized either with the schwar (e.g., /ɪɚ/) or with the consonantal /r/ (/ɪr/). The common rhotic diphthongs are:

Rhotic Diphthong	Example
/ɪr/	deer
/ɔr/	door
/ɑr/	dark
/ɛr/	dare
/ʊr/	poor

Pronunciations of these diphthongs vary depending on the speaker, the amount of stress on the word, and other factors. For example, it would not be unusual to hear the word *deer* pronounced as [dir] if it were said in isolation. In connected speech the vowels tend to be partially centralized, so the vowels used in the list are probably a better transcription. Also, in some dialects other diphthongs are present, and some distinctions are lost, as when the words *poor, pore,* and *pour* are all pronounced as [pɔr]. Work Exercise 7 to check understanding of diphthongs.

EXERCISE 7 ◇◇

DIRECTIONS: Indicate the diphthong found in each of the following words.

Word	Diphthong
1. joy	_____
2. how	_____
3. air	_____
4. show	_____
5. high	_____
6. now	_____
7. rode	_____
8. Roy	_____
9. mine	_____
10. save	_____
11. car	_____
12. store	_____
13. made	_____
14. beer	_____

◇◇

Syllable Structure Processes

Syllable structure processes are sound changes that affect the syllable shape of words. The change may be in the number of syllables produced or in the shape of the syllable (e.g., the arrangement of consonants and vowels or the deletion of a sound). Several processes fall under this category, including syllable deletion, reduplication, epenthesis, final-consonant deletion, initial-consonant deletion, cluster deletion, and cluster substitution.

Syllable Deletion

When a syllable of a polysyllabic word is omitted, that is called *syllable deletion*. Typically, the syllable deleted is unstressed. For this reason the process is sometimes labeled *weak syllable deletion* or *unstressed syllable deletion*. In connected speech, however, it is often difficult to determine the stress being placed on a particular syllable, so most assessment instruments will score any syllable omission as weak syllable deletion. For our purposes this process will be referred to as syllable deletion, defined as the omission of any syllable in the production of a polysyllabic word.

EXAMPLES: ——————————————————————————
telephone → [tɛlfon]
potato → [tedo]

Reduplication

The process of reduplication is defined as the partial or total repetition of a syllable of a word. This process is also referred to as *doubling*. In total reduplication, all of a syllable is repeated; whereas in partial reduplication, only part of the syllable (a consonant or a vowel) is repeated.

Reduplication usually affects multisyllabic words and appears to operate as a means of simplifying production. This process is included on the KLPA-2, HAPP-3, and SHAPE.

A special form of partial reduplication occurs when a final [i] is added to a word. This reduplication is referred to as *diminutization*.

EXAMPLES: ————————————————————————————————

Total: baby → [be be]

Partial: bottle → [ba da]

Diminutive: horse → [hɔrsi]

Epenthesis

Another process involving syllable change is epenthesis. In this process a sound (usually a vowel) is inserted between two consonants. The vowel that is typically inserted is the schwa. The SHAPE does not consider vowel insertion between consonants of a cluster as an error. Other types of epenthesis could be addition of a consonant or adding a vowel to the end of a word (Stoel-Gammon & Dunn, 1985). The insertion of the vowel adds another syllable to the target word and simplifies the production of the consonant cluster. Of the assessment instruments reviewed, only the HAPP-3 and SHAPE include epenthesis.

EXAMPLES: ————————————————————————————————

spoon → [səpun]

blue → [bəlu]

Final-Consonant Deletion

One of the easier processes to identify is final-consonant deletion. This process describes the deletion of a singleton consonant in word final position, resulting in an open syllable (e.g., CV). The CAAP and KLPA-2 include total cluster deletion as a form of final consonant deletion; however, for our purposes clusters will be treated as separate entities and will not be included under this process. On the HAPP-3, Hodson (2004) labeled this process *postvocalic singleton consonant omission*, defined as the deletion of a singleton consonant that terminates a syllable. The ALPHA–R includes this process in the category of "Consonant Deletion," along with initial-consonant deletion. The SHAPE restricts final-consonant deletion to obstruents.

EXAMPLES: ————————————————————————————————

skate → [ske]

peek → [pi]

baboon → [bæbu]

NOTE: Postvocalic /r/ and /l/ function more like vowels than consonants. As such, they are not typically considered when scoring for final-consonant deletion.

Initial-Consonant Deletion

Consonant deletion is not seen as commonly in word-initial position as it is in word-final. However, initial-consonant deletion does occur. It is defined as the deletion of a singleton consonant in word-initial position, resulting in the syllable's beginning with a vowel. Some definitions include the deletion of a cluster as an example of initial-consonant deletion (Khan & Lewis, 2002). As was the case with final-consonant deletion, we will treat clusters separately. On the HAPP-3 initial-consonant deletion is called *prevocalic singleton consonant omission,* defined as the deletion of a singleton consonant that initiates a syllable. The SHAPE treats initial-consonant deletion as an idiosyncratic process and also considers only consonant singletons.

EXAMPLES: _____

    team → [im]

    seat → [it]

    below → [ilo]

Cluster Deletion

Clusters, or blends, refer to adjacent consonants within a syllable. Cluster deletion is defined as the deletion of some (partial cluster deletion) or all of the consonants of a cluster. In partial cluster deletion, the segments deleted are typically those that are more difficult to produce.

EXAMPLES: _____

    Partial: stake → [teɪk]

    Total: stake → [eɪk]

    Partial: boats → [bot]

    Total: boats → [bo]

The SHAPE divides the clusters into categories: clusters with /w/, /l/, and /r/ and clusters with /s/. It also considers three element clusters separately. Hodson (2004) takes a slightly different approach to consonant sequences. On the HAPP-3 any consonant sequence (within or between syllables) falls under the heading of *consonant sequence reduction.* Most assessment instruments, however, look only at clusters within syllables, and that is the approach that will be used in this workbook. The CAAP calls the omission of one or more consonants from a two- or three-member cluster *cluster reduction.* If the entire cluster is omitted, it is scored as a deletion. Thus, in the word *most,* if the /st/ were omitted, it would be final consonant deletion on the CAAP, but cluster deletion on the ALPHA–R.

Cluster Substitution

Cluster substitution occurs when one member of a cluster is replaced with another consonant. Technically, this is not a syllable structure process, as the syllable number and shape remain intact. It is more properly a substitution process. It is presented here, however, in order to point out the contrast with cluster deletion. The cluster member substituted is typically the segment that is harder to produce and usually involves clusters made with liquids.

EXAMPLES:
blue → [bwu]
break → [bweɪk]

NOTE: Cluster deletion and cluster substitution are sometimes grouped together under the heading of *cluster reduction* or *cluster simplification* (BBTOP). Epenthesis might also be included under this heading, as it also simplifies the cluster structure.

Exercises 8 through 14 assist in developing understanding of syllable structure.

EXERCISE 10 ⬦⬦

DIRECTIONS: For each of the following words, determine if the child's production indicates total cluster deletion, partial cluster deletion, cluster substitution, or a combination.

Target	Child Form	Answer
1. blue	[bu]	_____
2. beast	[bi]	_____
3. glue	[gwu]	_____
4. spoon	[pun]	_____
5. tree	[twi]	_____
6. claw	[kɪ]	_____
7. skate	[eɪ]	_____
8. slow	[wo]	_____
9. plate	[pweɪt]	_____
10. straight	[tweɪt]	_____

EXERCISE 11

DIRECTIONS: For each of the following words, show the most likely effect of total cluster deletion, partial cluster deletion, and cluster substitution.

Target	Total Cluster Deletion	Partial Cluster Deletion	Cluster Substitution
1. play	_____	_____	_____
2. clay	_____	_____	_____
3. sleep	_____	_____	_____
4. break	_____	_____	_____
5. block	_____	_____	_____
6. strong	_____	_____	_____
7. prom	_____	_____	_____
8. creek	_____	_____	_____
9. grape	_____	_____	_____
10. string	_____	_____	_____

Note. It is typically the more difficult sounds that are deleted or substituted.

Substitution Processes

The majority of phonological processes involve some form of segment substitution that occurs independently of phonetic context (not due to assimilation). Keep in mind that the simple substitution of one segment for another does not define a phonological process. Processes involve a systematic sound change that affects classes of sounds or sound sequences. The replacement of a fricative with a stop is not a process when it occurs in isolation. If a *pattern* of stop substitutions for fricatives can be observed, however, then the sound change is identifiable as a phonological process.

This section of the workbook will define and provide exercises for the following substitution processes:

Stopping

Stridency Deletion

Fronting

Depalatalization

Palatalization

Affrication

Deaffrication

Backing

Alveolarization

Labialization

Gliding

Vowelization

Stopping

Several definitions of stopping (or *despirantization*) are available in the literature. The broadest definition describes stopping as the replacing of fricatives, affricates, liquids, or glides with a stop. The most common definition is the substitution of a stop for a fricative or affricate. When a stop replaces a liquid or glide, it is given the more specific label of stopping of liquids or stopping of glides.

The KLPA-2, SHAPE, and SPAT-D II define stopping as affecting fricatives and affricates, and that is the definition that will be used here. The SHAPE restricts evaluation of stopping to initial consonants. The BBTOP describes stopping as affecting fricatives and affricates but stipulates that it sometimes affects liquids as well. The ALPHA–R lists fricatives, affricates, liquids, and glides as sound classes that can be affected by stopping. The HAPP-3 defines stopping as the substitution of a stop consonant for a continuant phoneme. This definition leaves out affricates. Hodson (2004) questioned the definition of stopping, asking how an affricate can be made a stop when one of its components is already a stop. It might be argued, however, that processes typically describe the sound change that occurs and since the affricate class is being replaced by consonants from the stop class, the label *stopping* would therefore be appropriate.

Stopping can occur in all word positions, but in normally developing children it is more frequently seen in word-initial position than medially or finally (Dyson & Paden, 1983). The substitute stop usually has the same place feature as the target sound it replaces.

EXAMPLES:

    soap → [top]

    choke → [tok]

    feet → [pit]

Stridency Deletion

A process that often accompanies stopping is stridency deletion. Included on the HAPP-3, ALPHA–R, and SPAT-D II, this process is described as a sound change in which a strident consonant is either omitted or replaced with a nonstrident consonant. Perhaps the greatest difficulty in scoring stridency deletion is remembering which consonants are strident. Strident consonants are noisy consonants and include /f/, /v/, /s/, /z/, /ʃ/, /ʒ/, /ʧ/, and /ʤ/. Of the fricatives only /θ/, /ð/, and /h/ are not strident. Note that a frontal lisp, sometimes transcribed as /θ/, is actually a strident sound and not the nonstrident interdental.

EXAMPLES:

    soap → [θop]

    soap → [op]

    soap → [top]

Fronting

To understand fronting, the clinician must remember the places of articulation. In general, *fronting* means that the replacing sound has a more anterior place of articulation than the target sound. This, unfortunately, is too broad a definition. Fronting is more accurately the replacement of a back-of-the-mouth sound with a front sound. The boundary between front and back is the palatal-alveolar area just anterior to the rugae in the roof of the mouth. For the purposes of this workbook, we will describe fronting as occurring when sounds made in the back of the mouth (/k/, /g/, /ŋ/, /tʃ/, /dʒ/, /ʃ/, and /ʒ/) are replaced with sounds made anterior to the palatal area. The most common substitutions are alveolar stops.

The HAPP-3 does not score the sound change of palatals to alveolars as fronting because the place change is not considered major enough. Instead, this sound change is included in depalatalization. The BBTOP makes a distinction between fronting and depalatalization, with the latter being defined as the substitution of a palatal with a sound made in a position more forward in the mouth. The KLPA-2 and SPAT-D make a similar distinction but uses the labels *velar* and *palatal fronting*. The SHAPE describes fronting as the replacement of velars by alveolars.

EXAMPLES: ——————————————————————————————

  coat → [tout]

  show → [to] or [so]

  sing → [sin]

Depalatalization

This workbook makes a distinction between palatal fronting and depalatalization. The process of depalatalization occurs when a palatal sound is replaced with a nonpalatal sound. This process is also defined as movement of the place of articulation from the palatal position to a position more forward in the mouth (BBTOP). As such, it is sometimes referred to as *palatal fronting*. As used on the HAPP-3, the sound change can affect place or manner. The SHAPE divides this process into *depalatalization of initial singletons* and *depalatalization of final singletons*. The replacing sound must be a more anterior consonant. For this workbook, any sound change that replaces a palatal sound with a nonpalatal will be considered depalatalization.

EXAMPLES: ——————————————————————————————

  shoot → [sut] or [tut]

  chew → [su] or [tu]

NOTE: The change from a palatal to an alveolar is a minor shift in place of articulation. The major change that occurs to palatals is in sound production. The palatal sounds are made with the blade of the tongue, whereas the usual substitutions—/s/, /z/, /t/, and /d/—are all made with the tongue tip. This suggests that a more appropriate label for this sound change would be apicalization; however, none of the currently available phonology instruments uses this process description.

Palatalization

The process of palatalization is included on the HAPP-3 and describes the addition of a palatal component to a nonpalatal target phoneme.

EXAMPLES:
sew → [ʃo]
bees → [biʒ]

NOTE: Palatalization is sometimes included as an assimilatory process that occurs when nonpalatal consonants are followed by a glide or front vowel (Bernthal & Bankson, 1993).

EXAMPLE:
miss you → [miʃju]

Affrication

Affrication is included only on the ALPHA–R and the HAPP-3. This process involves the replacing of a fricative consonant with an affricate. Affrication is sometimes seen in children with a Spanish-language background. Bernthal and Bankson (1993) noted that /dʒ/ is an allophone of /j/, and [tʃ] is an allophone of /s/ in Spanish found in the baby-talk register.

EXAMPLES:
soap → [tʃop] or [tsop]
shoe → [tʃu]

Deaffrication

The process of deaffrication refers to the changing of an affricate to a stop or fricative. Some definitions limit the sound change to a fricative, but for our purposes any sound change that results in a nonaffricate will be considered deaffrication. This process is scored on the ALPHA–R, HAPP-3, KLPA-2, DEAP, and BBTOP.

EXAMPLES: ——————————————————————

    choose → [suz] or [tuz]

    jeep → [zip] or [dip]

    chain → [kem]

Backing

Backing is a process that is rare in normal phonological development. This process describes a sound change in which front consonants are replaced with back consonants (velars or glottals). Palatals are considered back on most distinctive feature systems, but for our purposes we will consider back sounds to include only velars or glottals. Thus a shift from a palatal to a velar or glottal placement would be considered backing. To help remember this, consider which part of the tongue is used in production. For velar sounds, the posterior part of the tongue is used; palatal productions use the tongue blade (anterior part of the tongue).

The SHAPE treats backing as an idiosyncratic process and divides it into *backing of initial alveolar consonants* and *backing of final alveolar consonants*. The replacement must be a velar.

Some instruments use more specific terminology. The term *glottalization* is used when the substitution is a glottal stop, and *velar backing* is used for velar substitution.

EXAMPLES: ——————————————————————

    shoe → [ku]

    dough → [go]

Alveolarization

The process of *alveolarization* has been narrowly defined as the replacing of consonants made with the lips or teeth with consonants made on the alveolar ridge. This process is used to explain such sound changes as /s/ for /f/ and /s/ for /θ/. Alveolarization is scored on the ALPHA–R and is referred to as a *place shift* on the HAPP-3.

EXAMPLES: ——————————————————————

    food → [sud]

    thin → [sɪn] or [tɪn]

Labialization

The process of *labialization* describes sound changes involving labial sounds replacing inter-dental or alveolar obstruents. The most common of these are [f] substituting for /θ/ and /v/ substituting for /ð/. The /l/ sound is not an obstruent and is thus not included in this sound change. The ALPHA–R is the only assessment instrument that includes this process. On the HAPP-3 this sound change is included under the category of *place shift*.

EXAMPLES:

sun → [fʌn]

thin → [fɪn]

NOTE: It is easy to confuse labialization with labial assimilation. The deciding factor is the presence or absence of other labials in the target word. If the sound change occurs in the absence of labial consonants in the target word, then the sound change is labialization. If the sound change occurs only in the presence of labial consonants, then the process is labial assimilation.

Gliding

Gliding is a very common process in the speech of children. This process describes the replacement of liquid consonants with glides. All of the assessment instruments reviewed for this workbook include the process of gliding. On the SHAPE it is called *gliding of initial liquids,* and the /h/ is considered a glide along with the /w/ and /j/. On the KLPA-2 liquid simplification includes both gliding and vowelization of liquids. A special form of gliding affects fricatives (sometimes affricates) and is referred to as *fricative (affricate) gliding.*

EXAMPLES:

road → [wod] or [jod]

low → [wo] or [jo]

Vowelization

When syllabic liquids or nasals are replaced with vowels, it is referred to as vowelization or vocalization. Although the /ɚ/ is considered a pure vowel, when it is centralized to a schwa or other pure vowel, it also is referred to as vowelization. The same is true for the various rhotic diphthongs. The most common vowel substitutions for the syllabics are [ə], [o], and [ʊ].

EXAMPLES:

table → [teɪbo]

bigger → [bɪgə]

car → [kə]

Exercises 15 through 20 provide practice in identifying subsitution processes.

EXERCISE 15 ◇◇

DIRECTIONS: For each of the following words, indicate whether stridency deletion, stopping, or both have occurred.

Target	Child Form	Process
Ex: save	[teɪv]	stopping, stridency deletion
1. soup	[tup]	_____
2. thin	[tɪn]	_____
3. base	[beɪt]	_____
4. house	[taʊf]	_____
5. moose	[mut]	_____
6. feet	[tit]	_____
7. zoo	[du]	_____
8. chase	[teɪs]	_____
9. shake	[teɪk]	_____
10. bath	[bæt]	_____

◇◇

⬦⬦⬦⬦⬦ EXERCISE 16 ⬦⬦⬦⬦⬦⬦⬦⬦⬦⬦⬦⬦⬦⬦⬦⬦⬦⬦⬦⬦⬦⬦⬦⬦⬦⬦⬦

DIRECTIONS: Determine which processes are possible for each of the following target words and place a check mark in the appropriate column(s).

Target Word	Stopping	Stridency Deletion	Fronting	Depalatalization	Palatalization	Affrication	Deaffrication
Ex: *suit*	✓	✓			✓	✓	
1. judge							
2. think							
3. kiss							
4. cheese							
5. sun							
6. moose							
7. case							
8. math							
9. shirt							
10. page							
11. path							
12. zoo							
13. ghost							
14. John							
15. face							

MINI-QUIZ 1 ◇◇◇

DIRECTIONS: Match the letter of each term to the correct definition or example.

a. reduplication

b. initial-consonant deletion

c. stopping

d. backing

e. labialization

f. partial

g. obstruents

h. deaffrication

i. gliding

j. fronting

k. weak

l. stridency deletion

m. final-consonant deletion

n. alveolarization

o. cluster deletion

p. labial

q. sonorants

r. palatalization

1. ___ process by which velars and palatals are replaced by alveolars

2. ___ type of reduplication that occurs when the two syllables are not identical

3. ___ process suggested by the deletion of an /s/, regardless of word position

4. ___ process by which labials or interdentals are replaced by alveolar sounds

5. ___ process that affects both of the liquids

6. ___ EX: /stov/ becoming [tov]

7. ___ process suggested by the replacement of an /s/ with a /ʃ/

8. ___ group that includes nasals, glides, and liquids

9. ___ syllable typically deleted in syllable deletion

10. ___ process suggested by the replacement of /tʃ/ with /s/

11. ___ category made up of the fricatives, affricates, and stops

12. ___ EX: /bot/ changing to [ot]

13. ___ EX: /to/ changing to [ko]

14. ___ place in which /w/, /p/, and /f/ are produced

◇◇

Assimilation Processes

Mackay (1987) defined assimilation as the phenomenon whereby a sound becomes more like a neighboring sound. Assimilation, also called *consonant harmony,* occurs when changes in speech production can be attributed to the influence of the phonetic context. These changes can affect place, manner, and/or voicing of speech sounds. To understand assimilation, keep in mind that in a phonetic context (e.g., a word) where assimilation occurs, there is a sound that changes and a sound that influences (causes) the change. The relationship between these two sounds helps us describe the assimilation.

Assimilation can be regressive or progressive. If the changing sound precedes the one that influences it, the change is called *regressive* or *anticipatory.* If a sound changes to become more like a sound it follows, it is called *progressive assimilation,* because the characteristics of the affecting sound have "progressed" into a following sound. Of the two, regressive assimilation is more commonly seen in children learning to speak American English.

Of the common phonology assessment instruments, only the SHAPE scores regressive and progressive assimilation. Regressive assimilation is defined as occurring when the initial consonant is replaced by a consonant that is similar in place, manner, or voicing or is the same as another consonant in the word. Progressive assimilation occurs when the final consonant is replaced by a consonant that is similar in place, manner, or voicing or is the same as another consonant in the word.

Assimilatory changes can be partial or total. If a sound changes so that it is identical to the influencing sound, then the assimilation is considered *total.* If only some of the features change to make the sound more like the influencing segment, then the assimilation is called *partial.*

Finally, assimilation can also be described by the presence or absence of intervening sounds. If there is no intervening sound between the changed segment and the influencing segment, the environment is called *contiguous.* If there is an intervening segment, then the assimilatory environment is *noncontiguous.* For example, the word *blue* might change to [bwu].

The /l/ sound is influenced by the adjacent labial, /b/, and becomes the labial /w/. As there are no intervening sounds between /b/ and /l/, this is an example of a contiguous environment.

EXAMPLES:

    gate → [tet] total, noncontiguous

    gate →[det] partial, noncontiguous

    blue →[bwu] partial, contiguous

Unlike the other phonological processes presented thus far, potential assimilatory processes cannot be identified based on sound changes occurring in a single word. Instead, several of the child's responses must be examined to determine if assimilation is occurring. Assimilation refers to sound changes that occur due to the influence of phonetic context, but to determine this, one must look at other contexts. Put simply, the sound changes occur only in given environments and not elsewhere. To "prove" assimilation, the clinician must identify the environments that control the sound change.

EXAMPLE:

Target	Child Form
she	[ʃi]
sheet	[tit]
shoe	[ʃu]
shoot	[tut]
shape	[tep]

In the preceding example, the child is not consistent in his or her substitutions. In some cases a /t/ replaces the /ʃ/, and at other times the target sound is correctly produced. By examining the phonetic environments, we find that the sound change to a stop occurs only in the presence of other stops (/t/ and /p/). Otherwise, the child produces the target sound correctly. This example would be a strong argument for assimilation. In some environments the sound change occurs, and in other environments the sound change is absent. In other words, context influences the production.

It helps to keep in mind that for assimilation to occur there must be something to assimilate to. The clinician's task is to discover what is influencing the sound change. This is a valuable skill to develop, because it helps the clinician to narrowly define the phonological system used by the child in his or her attempts to produce the adult target.

As noted, in identifying assimilation it is important to determine the environments that trigger sound change. Assimilation might be influenced by vowel height, manner of articulation, place of articulation, voicing, or some combination of these factors. One of the difficulties in identifying assimilation is that it may not occur all of the time. In the workbook exercises, assimilation will occur 100% of the time to help the clinician learn the basics, but in practice, the assimilation may occur inconsistently.

Common Forms of Assimilation

Labial Assimilation

Edwards and Shriberg (1983) described *labial assimilation* as a process in which a consonant in a word becomes a labial due to the influence of another labial consonant. The key to its identification is the presence of a labial consonant. If a labial is not present in the environment, then labial assimilation is not a possibility.

EXAMPLES: ————————————————————————————
table → [bebo]
rob → [wɑb]

NOTE: Assimilatory changes may be influenced by substitutions made in the production of words. For example, the child might make a w/r substitution, thus adding a labial component to the context that was not in the original target word (tree → [twi] → [pwi]).

Alveolar Assimilation

This process occurs when a sound in a word assimilates to an alveolar segment located elsewhere in the word.

EXAMPLES: ————————————————————————————
goat → [dot]
goat → [tot]
feet → [tit]

Velar Assimilation

This assimilation, also called *back assimilation,* occurs when a sound in a word becomes more like a velar sound located elsewhere in the word. The clinician must be careful not to confuse back assimilation with the process of backing.

EXAMPLES:

dog → [gɔg]

cot → [kɔg]

take → [keɪk]

Nasal Assimilation

Nasal assimilation occurs when a sound becomes more like a nasal consonant located nearby in the phonetic context.

EXAMPLES:

van → [næn]

window → [mɪndo]

NOTE: Nasal, labial, velar, and alveolar assimilations are all included on the HAPP-3 and SHAPE. The KLPA-2 and BBTOP use the general category of consonant harmony to cover all of the above assimilations.

Prevocalic Voicing

Prevocalic voicing occurs when voiceless obstruents preceding vowels become voiced. This is sometimes considered to be an assimilation to the voicing feature of the following vowel.

EXAMPLES:

pea → [di]

take → [deɪk]

cake → [geɪk]

Postvocalic Devoicing

This process results when a voiced obstruent in word-final position becomes voiceless. Like prevocalic voicing, this process is sometimes considered to be assimilatory. In this case the assimilation is to the voiceless feature of the following word boundary.

EXAMPLES:

rag → [ræk]

made → [met]

NOTE: Prevocalic voicing and postvocalic devoicing are evaluated by the KLPA-2 and DEAP. The ALPHA–R uses the label voicing change, and the HAPP-3 scores these changes under voicing alterations. The SHAPE looks only at the prevocalic position, calling it voicing of initial voiceless consonants.

Metathesis

Hodson and Paden (1991) defined *metathesis* as a process in which there is a reversal of the position of two sounds. The sounds need not be adjacent to one another, nor do they have to occur in the same word.

EXAMPLES: ————————————————————————————————

ask → [æks]

boast → [bots]

Coalescence

To coalesce means to collapse or combine into a whole. In the process of *coalescence,* features of two adjacent segments are collapsed to form one segment with features from both of the original segments.

EXAMPLES: ————————————————————————————————

spoon → [fun]

train → [fen]

In the first example the /sp/ was replaced with an /f/. The /f/ has the fricative feature from the /s/ and the labial feature from the /p/.

Khan (1985) indicated that coalescence can occur for syllables as well. In this form, two syllables are collapsed into one syllable, which has segments from both (e.g., button → [bʌn]). In this workbook, however, we will deal only with changes within one syllable.

NOTE: The processes of coalescence and metathesis are included on the HAPP-3 and the KLPA-2.

Work Exercises 21 through 28 to further your understanding of forms of assimilation.

<<<<<<<<<< **EXERCISE 21** <<<<<<<<<<<<<<<<<<<<<<<<<<<<<<<<<<<<<<<<<<<<<<<<<<<<<<<<<<<<<

DIRECTIONS: For each word in the list below, determine if the indicated assimilation is progressive or regressive, contiguous or noncontiguous.

Target	Child Form	Answer
Ex: *soap*	[pop]	regressive, noncontiguous
1. coat	[tot]	_____
2. take	[teɪt]	_____
3. suit	[zut]	_____
4. cat	[kæk]	_____
5. sheet	[sit]	_____
6. face	[feɪf]	_____
7. room	[wum]	_____
8. shake	[keɪk]	_____
9. break	[bweɪk]	_____
10. tack	[tæt]	_____
11. goat	[gok]	_____
12. lame	[weɪm]	_____
13. sad	[tæd]	_____
14. safe	[feɪf]	_____
15. thumb	[fʌm]	_____

<<<<<<<<<<<<<<<<<<<<<<<<<<<<<<<<<<<<<<<<<<<<<<<<<<<<<<<<<<<<<<<<<<<<<<<<<<<<<<<<<<<<<<<<<<

EXERCISE 22 ◇◇

DIRECTIONS: For each of the following words, determine if the sound change might be due to assimilation. Remember, in assimilation, a sound changes to become more like another sound in the same word.

Target Word	Child Form	Sound Change	Assimilation Maybe	No
Ex: *coat*	[tot]	k → t	X	
coat	[kod]	t → d		X
1. take	[teɪt]	k → t	_____	_____
2. lame	[deɪm]	l → d	_____	_____
3. sheet	[tit]	ʃ → t	_____	_____
4. tape	[keɪp]	t → k	_____	_____
5. tip	[kɪp]	t → k	_____	_____
6. case	[seɪs]	k → s	_____	_____
7. tack	[tæg]	k → g	_____	_____
8. shake	[geɪk]	ʃ → g	_____	_____
9. face	[veɪs]	f → v	_____	_____
10. leaf	[wif]	l → w	_____	_____

◇◇

EXERCISE 23

DIRECTIONS: Examine the following words and underline those in which prevocalic voicing could occur.

shoe	bad	patch
cake	thumb	kitty
got	coat	bye-bye
chips	run	candy
sock	fun	that

EXERCISE 24

DIRECTIONS: Examine the following words and underline those in which postvocalic devoicing could occur.

this	pad	pitch
nose	save	half
rub	cot	leash
lid	bike	have
judge	kid	rose

EXERCISE 25 ◇◇

DIRECTIONS: For each of the following words, determine if the sound change(s) indicates the possibility of prevocalic voicing (PrV), postvocalic devoicing (PDe), both, or neither.

Target Word	Child Form	Sound Change	PrV	PDe	Neither
Ex: *tape*	[deɪp]	t → d	X		
1. robe	[rop]	b → p			
2. two	[du]	t → d			
3. seed	[dit]	s → d d → t			
4. made	[meɪt]	d → t			
5. sad	[tæd]	s → t			
6. page	[peɪs]	ʤ → s			
7. Sue	[du]	s → d			
8. nose	[not]	z → t			
9. toad	[dot]	t → d d → t			
10. safe	[teɪp]	s → t f → p			

◇◇

EXERCISE 26

DIRECTIONS: Examine the words in the list below. Write whether each one has undergone coalescence or metathesis.

Target	Child Form	Answer
1. tree	[fi]	_____
2. host	[hots]	_____
3. ask	[æks]	_____
4. behave	[hibeɪv]	_____
5. star	[tʃɑr]	_____
6. most	[mots]	_____
7. spoon	[fun]	_____
8. trick	[fɪk]	_____
9. tea cup	[kitʌp]	_____
10. spark	[fɑrk]	_____

EXERCISE 27 ◇◇◇

DIRECTIONS: In each of the following words, a target sound is underlined. Determine which forms of assimilation are possible should a substitution be made for the target. *Hint: Compare place and manner features of the target sound and the influencing consonant.*

Target	Labial	Alveolar	Velar	Nasal
Ex: <u>sh</u>oot	_____	X	_____	_____
1. <u>l</u>imb	_____	_____	_____	_____
2. <u>t</u>ake	_____	_____	_____	_____
3. <u>f</u>arm	_____	_____	_____	_____
4. ga<u>t</u>e	_____	_____	_____	_____
5. <u>c</u>an	_____	_____	_____	_____
6. ba<u>k</u>e	_____	_____	_____	_____
7. <u>l</u>ine	_____	_____	_____	_____
8. <u>l</u>oop	_____	_____	_____	_____
9. <u>d</u>og	_____	_____	_____	_____
10. <u>ch</u>eese	_____	_____	_____	_____

◇◇◇

◇◇◇◇◇◇◇◇◇ **EXERCISE 28** ◇◇◇

DIRECTIONS: For each of the following words, indicate whether the sound change is indicative of labial, alveolar, velar, and/or nasal assimilation.

Target	Child Form	Sound Change	Labial	Alveolar	Velar	Nasal
Ex: *rope*	[wop]	r → w	X			
1. take	[keɪk]					
2. game	[meɪm]					
3. cone	[ton]					
4. coat	[kok]					
5. shoot	[tut]					
6. win	[mɪn]					
7. save	[feɪv]					
8. soap	[pop]					
9. loaf	[wof]					
10. goat	[dot]					
11. dog	[gɔg]					
12. thief	[fif]					

◇◇◇

Determining Assimilation

As noted, it is not possible to determine assimilation from a single sound change. Phonetic contexts must be compared to confirm that the sound changes occur only in particular environments. It is best to approach this task in steps. Examine the following speech sample:

Target	Child Form		Target	Child Form
1. shoot	[tut]		6. fat	[pæt]
2. seat	[tit]		7. suit	[tut]
3. far	[far]		8. shoe	[ʃu]
4. cheat	[tit]		9. see	[si]
5. cheese	[ʧiz]		10. Sue	[su]

Step One

Determine the sound changes that take place. Enter them in the space provided below:

You should have noted the following substitutions: t/s, t/ʧ, p/f, and t/ʃ.

Step Two

Determine if there is variability in the sound substitutions. Examine the sample for inconsistencies. Are there word contexts in which the sounds are made correctly? Enter your findings below:

The sample contains instances of each of the target sounds being produced correctly and incorrectly. Inconsistency in sound production can signal the presence of assimilation.

Step Three

Look for similarities within the environments in which the sounds are made correctly to distinguish between the environments in which sound changes occur. Where sound changes occur can you find an influencing sound that would account for the change? Can you find any commonalities in either group? Try to find minimal-pair words produced for the target sound in which one word has the sound change and the other does not. Enter your findings in the space provided:

For this rather contrived speech sample, the targets change to stops only in the presence of stop consonants. Word pairs like *Sue–suit* and *cheese–cheat* supply the evidence. The two words in a pair have the same targets, but only the words *suit* and *cheat* are produced with substitutions. This yields a working hypothesis for assimilation: Fricatives and affricates change to stops in the presence of stops.

Step Four

The final step is to confirm your hypothesis. Reexamine the speech sample. Do the sound changes occur only in environments where there are stop consonants in the target word? Are the targets produced differently in words without stop consonants? If this is the case (and it certainly is for this limited sample), then you have "proven" assimilation—in this case, assimilation to manner (stop-plosives).

> NOTE: Remember, although we have practiced identifying only labial, velar alveolar, and nasal assimilation, the sound changes in assimilation can be to any place, manner, and/or voicing and even to vowel height.

Another consideration in determining assimilation is word position. Some sound changes are position sensitive. Good examples are prevocalic voicing and postvocalic devoicing. Word position is also important in determining whether the assimilations are regressive or progressive in nature. Remember, regressive assimilations are sound changes that typically affect consonants beginning a word, while progressive assimilations affect consonants near or in word-final position. In the given examples, all of the assimilations are regressive.

In Exercises 29 and 30, determine whether assimilation exists in the speech samples provided.

EXERCISE 29 ◇◇

DIRECTIONS: Below is a representative speech sample of a 4-year-old child. Only the words relevant to making a decision about assimilation have been provided. Examine the sound changes and try to determine a working hypothesis about the presence or absence of assimilation. *Hint: Look for minimal or near-minimal pairs.*

Target	Child Form	Target	Child Form
1. Kay	[ke]	6. goat	[dot]
2. gate	[det]	7. go	[go]
3. sheet	[tit]	8. Joe	[dʒo]
4. Jane	[deɪn]	9. she	[ʃi]
5. kite	[taɪt]	10. Gay	[ge]

Sound changes:

Inconsistencies:

Working hypothesis:

◇◇

EXERCISE 30

DIRECTIONS: Below is another speech sample. This time some irrelevant sound changes have been included to make the task a bit more difficult. Try to determine a working hypothesis about the presence or absence of assimilation.

Target	Child Form	Target	Child Form
1. farm	[fɑrm]	7. dart	[dɑrt]
2. two	[tu]	8. back	[gæk]
3. took	[kʊk]	9. do	[du]
4. dog	[gɔg]	10. take	[kek]
5. dark	[gɑrk]	11. baby	[beɪbɪ]
6. tag	[kæg]	12. top	[tɔp]

Sound changes:

Inconsistencies:

Working hypothesis:

Differentiating From Other Processes

Assimilations can easily be confused with other phonological processes. For example, velar assimilation might be mistaken for backing, and fronting might be confused with alveolar assimilation. The differentiating characteristic to look for is consistency. When assimilation is present, there will be a variable substitution pattern that is a function of the phonetic context. The other processes operate independently: Context is not a factor in their occurrence.

As a general rule, therefore, if you can determine that sound changes are dependent on the presence of a particular context, the process is assimilation. If context is irrelevant, then you are dealing with another type of phonological process. Try Exercises 31 to 34 to determine whether sound changes are due to assimilation or another process.

EXERCISE 31 ◇◇◇

DIRECTIONS: Examine the following responses and determine if alveolar assimilation is occurring or if the sound changes are due simply to fronting and stopping, without any assimilation effect.

Target	Child Form		Target	Child Form
1. shoot	[tut]		6. sheet	[tit]
2. case	[teɪt]		7. Jeep	[dip]
3. she	[ti]		8. goose	[dut]
4. go	[do]		9. Sue	[tu]
5. far	[fɑr]		10. suit	[tut]

Conclusion:

Reasoning:

EXERCISE 32

DIRECTIONS: Examine the words listed below and determine whether velar assimilation is occurring.

Target	Child Form	Target	Child Form
1. take	[keɪk]	5. toe	[to]
2. back	[gæk]	6. talk	[kɔk]
3. top	[tɑp]	7. shake	[kek]
4. bow	[bo]	8. sheet	[tit]

Conclusion:

Reasoning:

EXERCISE 33 ◇◇◇

DIRECTIONS: Examine the following sample and determine whether the sound changes are due to labialization or labial assimilation.

Target	Child Form	Target	Child Form
1. thin	[tɪn]	6. thumb	[fʌm]
2. those	[doz]	7. the	[di]
3. them	[vɛm]	8. some	[fʌm]
4. sun	[sʌn]	9. see	[si]
5. safe	[feɪf]	10. same	[feɪm]

Conclusion:

Reasoning:

◇◇

DIRECTIONS: Examine the following sample and determine whether the sound changes are due to stopping or alveolar assimilation.

Target	Child Form	Target	Child Form
1. cake	[teɪt]	6. goat	[dot]
2. shoe	[tu]	7. shoot	[tut]
3. go	[do]	8. key	[ti]
4. cheat	[tit]	9. Joe	[do]
5. show	[to]	10. Kay	[te]

Conclusion:

Reasoning:

◇◇

A Final Note

You should have had no difficulty differentiating between assimilation and other processes in the exercises. Reality could be a different story, however, as the assimilatory influence might not operate all of the time. In such cases, you would find exceptions to your hypothesis. In rule-writing terminology, variable assimilations would be described as *optional,* whereas invariable assimilations would be termed *obligatory.* The problem is that the child's system is changing, with any number of influences operating at any one time.

So when is the term *assimilation* appropriate? If analysis shows that the sound changes occur only in a given environment (even if not 100% of the time), then the process is assimilation. The key is that the particular sound changes do not occur in other environments. Thus it is quite possible that a child might substitute /t/ for /k/ only when alveolars are present elsewhere in the word but make that substitution in only half of the words fitting that description. If that is the only environment where the sound change occurs, the process is still assimilation.

The assessment instruments currently available are not designed to guide the clinician through an analysis for assimilation. Instead, they function to alert the clinician to the possibility of assimilation by identifying sound changes that could be attributed to phonetic context. The clinician must take the initiative and compare the sound changes in those contexts with sounds in other contexts to determine if assimilation is actually occurring.

In many cases the sample from the assessment instrument will be too limited for comparison. The clinician must then do extension testing using minimal- and near-minimal-pair word stimuli to help prove a case for or against assimilation. Once again, if the sound change occurs in contexts without an influencing sound, then the sound change is not due to assimilation. Proving assimilation requires that the sound changes occur *only* in environments in which the target sound becomes more like another sound elsewhere in the word.

CHAPTER 5

Vowel Processes

The study of children's phonological disorders has traditionally focused on consonantal errors. Studies by Pollock and Keiser (1990) and Stoel-Gammon (1990) opened the door to the study of vowel misarticulations, including potential vowel processes.

Vowel processes are two or more segmental errors that can be accounted for by the same rule (Pollock, 1994). Of the assessment instruments reviewed for this text, only the ALPHA–R includes procedures for evaluating for vowel processes. Pollock proposed dividing the vowel error patterns into three categories: (a) feature changes, (b) complexity changes, and (c) vowel harmony. "Feature change patterns involve the substitution or merging of one or more of the vowel features of height, frontness, tenseness, or lip rounding. Complexity change patterns involve diphthongization of monophthongs. Vowel harmony patterns involve errors in multisyllabic words where one vowel changes in order to share one or more features with another vowel in the word" (p. 30).

In determining the processes, the examiner compares the vowel error with its target in terms of the vowel features, complexity, or similarity of features. Thus the examiner needs to be familiar with the vowel quadrangle and be able to differentiate between diphthongs and monophthongs.

Following are brief definitions of the vowel processes assessed by the ALPHA–R, some of which are taken from Pollock and Keiser (1990). As with consonantal processes, the name of the process describes the sound change. These definitions are followed by Exercises 35 through 37.

Vowel Backing

A vowel is replaced with a more posterior vowel.

EXAMPLE: _____

bit → [but]

Vowel Lowering

A vowel is replaced with a vowel made with a lower tongue position.

EXAMPLE: _____

beet → [bɪt]

Vowel Raising

A vowel is replaced with a vowel made with a higher tongue position.

EXAMPLE: _____

bat → [bet]

Centralization

A vowel is replaced by a vowel with a more central tongue position.

EXAMPLE: _____

boat → [bʌt]

Vowel Unrounding

A normally rounded vowel is replaced with a nonrounded vowel.

EXAMPLE: _____

boat → [bɑt]

Diphthongization

A monophthong vowel is produced as a diphthong.

EXAMPLE: _____

bet → [bɛɪt]

Diphthong Reduction

A diphthong is produced as a monophthong.

EXAMPLE: _____

Mike → [mɑk]

Complete Vowel Harmony

One vowel is changed so that two vowels in a word are the same. Vowels can also assimilate to tenseness or height.

EXAMPLES: _____

coffee → [kifi]

office → [ɔfɔs]

EXERCISE 35 ⬦⬦⬦⬦⬦⬦⬦⬦⬦⬦⬦⬦⬦⬦⬦⬦⬦⬦⬦⬦⬦⬦⬦⬦⬦⬦⬦⬦⬦⬦⬦⬦⬦⬦⬦⬦

DIRECTIONS: For each of the following target vowels, underline the vowels that are raised, backed, or lowered in comparison. Some changes will not apply, and some will have more than one correct answer.

Target	Raised	Backed	Lowered
ɪ	o i e	e o i	o i e
o	e ɛ u	u ɪ e	e ɛ ɔ
e	ɪ æ u	ɔ i ɪ	u ɪ ɛ
ʌ	u æ ɑ	o i e	ɪ æ o
æ	ɑ e u	ɪ e ʊ	ɑ e u
ɛ	ɪ æ o	ɪ æ u	ɔ ɪ ɑ
i	u ɪ e	e ɛ u	u ɔ ɛ
u	e ɑ i	u æ ɑ	ɪ æ o
ɔ	u æ ɑ	ɑ e u	ɪ æ u
ɚ	ɪ æ u	ɪ æ o	ɪ ʌ ʊ

⬦⬦

⬦⬦⬦⬦⬦⬦ EXERCISE 36 ⬦⬦⬦⬦⬦⬦⬦⬦⬦⬦⬦⬦⬦⬦⬦⬦⬦⬦⬦⬦⬦⬦⬦⬦⬦⬦⬦⬦⬦⬦⬦⬦⬦

DIRECTIONS: Below is a list of bisyllabic target words with two vowels each. Determine what the second vowel of each word would be in the cases of complete vowel harmony, tenseness harmony, and height harmony. Underline the correct answers.

Target	Complete	Tenseness	Height
Ci C<u>ɛ</u>	o ɪ i	ɛ e ɑ	ɛ u ɑ
Cɑ C<u>o</u>	e ɑ æ	ʊ ɛ i	ɝ ɪ u
Ce C<u>ɪ</u>	ɔ ɛ e	ɛ ʊ æ	u ɛ o
Cu C<u>ʊ</u>	ɔ ɪ u	ɛ ə o	e i ɑ
Co C<u>ɪ</u>	o æ i	ɛ e ɑ	æ e ɑ
Cæ C<u>ɪ</u>	e ɑ æ	o ʊ ɛ	ɑ u i
Cu C<u>ə</u>	ɑ ə u	æ ɪ e	ɛ i æ
Cæ C<u>ɪ</u>	æ ɪ u	ʊ e ɔ	ɛ e ɑ

⬦⬦⬦⬦⬦⬦ EXERCISE 37 ⬦⬦⬦⬦⬦⬦⬦⬦⬦⬦⬦⬦⬦⬦⬦⬦⬦⬦⬦⬦⬦⬦⬦⬦⬦⬦⬦⬦⬦⬦⬦⬦⬦

DIRECTIONS: In each row of the table, underline the vowel or vowels that fit the description to the left: rounded, tense, lax, or diphthong.

Rounded	ɪ	e	oʊ	ɑ	u
Tense	ɛ	oʊ	u	ɪ	i
Diphthong	e	u	ɑʊ	æ	ɔɪ
Lax	u	e	ɪ	ɔ	i
Rounded	e	ʊ	ɔ	ʌ	æ
Tense	ʌ	ʊ	æ	e	oʊ
Diphthong	ɛr	ɑ	oʊ	ɑɪ	i

MINI-QUIZ 2 ◇◇◇

DIRECTIONS: Match the letter of each term to the correct definition or example.

a. regressive
b. contiguous
c. alveolar assimilation
d. backing
e. labialization
f. coalescence
g. vowel raising
h. diphthongization
i. vowel backing

j. progressive
k. total
l. labial assimilation
m. velar assimilation
n. alveolarization
o. metathesis
p. monophthong
q. centralization
r. vowel lowering

1. _____ process that might be occurring if /e/ is replaced by /o/
2. _____ type of assimilation that occurs when the sound that changes occurs first
3. _____ type of assimilation that has a sound change affected by /k/ or /g/
4. _____ process that might be confused with labial assimilation
5. _____ process that might be occurring if /ɪ/ is replaced by /æ/
6. _____ EX: /sef/ becoming [fef]
7. _____ process that might be occurring if /e/ is replaced by /ʌ/
8. _____ type of assimilation that occurs when the changing sound and the influencing sound become exactly alike
9. _____ EX: /ɑ/ becoming [ɑɪ]
10. _____ EX: /spun/ becoming [fun]
11. _____ process that might be confused with velar assimilation
12. _____ EX: /kot/ changing to [tot]
13. _____ EX: /wɪsk/ changing to [wɪks]
14. _____ term used to describe a changing sound and an influencing sound side by side

◇◇◇

Distinctive Features

Distinctive features are considered the smallest indivisible units that make up phonemes. When produced together, these units form speech sounds. You might think of features as notes that make up a musical chord. Each note has its own quality, but when it is played with other notes, together they form a unique sound—a chord. In terms of speech, distinctive features are typically described by their acoustic or articulatory characteristics and presented in a binary system. For example, the feature [nasal] refers to sounds in which air passes through the nasal cavity. Phonemes that have this feature are designated as being [+ nasal], and phonemes made without air passing through the nose are [− nasal]. Each phoneme can be described as a bundle of particular features, just as each chord can be described as a combination of particular notes played at one time.

The features that are important to differentiating the phonemes of a language are called distinctive features. The feature of voicing is distinctive in English. As seen in our review of place, manner, and voicing (see Chapter 1), the phonemes /t/ and /d/ share the same place and manner but differ in voicing. The /t/ has the feature [− voice] and the /d/ has the feature [+ voice]. In contrast, the feature of aspiration is not distinctive in English. A /t/ sound can be made with or without aspiration and still be recognized as /t/. In Hindi, however, aspiration is distinctive because the presence or absence of aspiration determines what phoneme is produced. A distinctive feature system will have enough features so that there is at least one feature difference between any two phonemes. In other words, each phoneme will have a unique bundle of features that differs from that of every other phoneme by at least one feature.

The value of features is that phonemes can be compared to one another based on the features they share or don't share. The thought is that if a child misarticulates several speech sounds that share a common feature, intervention that focuses on facilitating the development of that feature should result in improved articulation of all of the error sounds. Features have also been used in target selection with intervention programs using minimal and maximal oppositions. Some evidence suggests that children with multiple articulation errors will demonstrate greater generalization when the treatment uses maximal oppositions (Gierut, 1990). Finally, distinctive features are often the basis on which phonological theories are proposed and tested.

Many distinctive feature systems have been described. Jakobson, Fant, and Halle (1952) proposed an early system that used twelve acoustic features. Chomsky and Halle (1968) proposed a later system that has had considerable application to the field of speech–language pathology. Other systems have been developed, each with its own strengths and weaknesses. Rather than attempt to present several distinctive feature systems, this workbook will focus on familiarizing the student with some of the more common consonant features shared by the various systems. The following features will be addressed in this chapter: sonorant, obstruent, continuant, voice, nasal, strident, labial, coronal, and back. A summary of the features associated with the English consonants is displayed in Table 4.

Sonorant

The feature of [sonorant] refers to a manner of speech production that allows the vocal folds to vibrate spontaneously without a rise in air pressure above the level of the larynx. In other words, the vocal tract is open enough so that no special adjustments of the larynx are needed in order to initiate voicing. Sonorancy is considered by Chomsky and Halle (1968) to be a major class feature, meaning that it can be used to divide the speech sounds into broader categories of other sound classes. The sonorant sounds include the liquids, glides, and nasals (and vowels). Sonorant sounds are those that are regularly voiced. Bernhardt and Stemberger (2000) include the /h/ sound and the glottal stop (ʔ) as sonorants, both of which are voiceless. These sounds would qualify because the subglottic air pressure is low and would not cause a rise in the air pressure above the level of the larynx.

TABLE 4

Distinctive Feature Matrix Based on Common Definitions of Features

Distinctive Features	p	b	t	d	k	g	tʃ	dʒ	f	v	θ	ð	s	z	ʃ	ʒ	h	w	j	l	r	m	n	ŋ
Sonorant	−	−	−	−	−	−	−	−	−	−	−	−	−	−	−	−	−	+	+	+	+	+	+	+
Obstruent	+	+	+	+	+	+	+	+	+	+	+	+	+	+	+	+	+	−	−	−	−	−	−	−
Continuant	−	−	−	−	−	−	−	−	+	+	+	+	+	+	+	+	+	+	+	+	+	−	−	−
Voice	−	+	−	+	−	+	−	+	−	+	−	+	−	+	−	+	−	+	+	+	+	+	+	+
Nasal	−	−	−	−	−	−	−	−	−	−	−	−	−	−	−	−	−	−	−	−	−	+	+	+
Strident	−	−	−	−	−	−	+	+	+	+	−	−	+	+	+	+	−	−	−	−	−	−	−	−
Labial	+	+	−	−	−	−	−	−	+	+	−	−	−	−	−	−	−	+	−	−	+	+	−	−
Coronal	−	−	+	+	−	−	+	+	−	−	+	+	+	+	+	+	−	−	−	+	+	−	+	−
Back	−	−	−	−	+	+	−	−	−	−	−	−	−	−	−	−	−	+	−	−	−	−	−	+

Obstruent

Obstruents are speech sounds that are produced with considerable constriction, so that voicing would not occur unless there were special adjustments of the vocal folds. Obstruency can be considered another major class, as it also divides the speech sounds into broad categories. Obstruents include stops, affricates, and fricatives (sound classes that have voiceless members).

Research by Gierut (1990, 1992) suggests that choosing opposition pairs that cross major class boundaries results in greater generalization when compared to working with opposition pairs from the same class. Thus if a child had errors with the following sounds: /r/, /l/, /s/, /ʃ/, /tʃ/, and /dʒ/, an opposition pair like *shoot–root* might result in greater generalization than the pair, *shoot–suit*. In the first pair, the /ʃ/ is an obstruent and the /r/ a sonorant; whereas, in the /s/ and /ʃ/ pair, both are from the obstruent class.

Complete Exercise 38, which provides practice in recognizing major class distinctions.

EXERCISE 38 ◇◇◇

DIRECTIONS: For the following sound pairs, determine whether the opposition crosses major classes (one is a sonorant and one is an obstruent) or the sounds are from the same sound class.

Sound Pair	Cross Major Classes?	
1. /s/-/r/	Yes	No
2. /n/-/l/	Yes	No
3. /t/-/h/	Yes	No
4. /m/-/h/	Yes	No
5. /z/-/f/	Yes	No
6. /j/-/g/	Yes	No
7. /tʃ/-/d/	Yes	No
8. /v/-/g/	Yes	No
9. /θ/-/ŋ/	Yes	No
10. /ʒ/-/ð/	Yes	No
11. /ʃ/-/dʒ/	Yes	No
12. /j/-/dʒ/	Yes	No

◇◇

Continuant

The feature of continuancy refers to a manner of production in which the airstream continues to move through the oral cavity. Continuants include glides, liquids, and fricatives. Nasals are not considered continuants because in their case the airstream is directed through the nasal cavity not the oral cavity. Common continuant speech errors involve fricatives and liquids. Thus the feature of continuancy is often considered an important feature for children to master.

Voice

The voice feature is associated with the same sounds as noted in the place-manner-voicing chart covered in Chapter 1 (Table 3). Voicing refers to vocal fold vibration during the production of the speech sound. All nasals, liquids, and glides are voiced. In addition, the stops, fricatives, and affricates also have voiced members. Sounds with the [+ voice] feature: /b/, /d/, /g/, /v/, /ð/, /z/, /ʒ/, /dʒ/, /m/, /n/, /ŋ/, /l/, /r/, /w/, and /j/. All of the other speech sounds (consonants) in English are considered [− voice].

Nasal

Sounds made with the airstream directed through the nasal cavity have the feature [+ nasal]. Nasal sounds are made with an open velopharyngeal port. They include: /m/, /n/, /ŋ/. The glides, liquids, and obstruents are considered [− nasal].

Strident

The characteristic of stridency was mentioned previously in the definition of the stridency deletion process in Chapter 3. Strident sounds are noisy sounds and include both fricatives and affricates. Some fricatives are noisier than others, so not all fricatives are [+ strident]. Of the nine fricatives, all are strident except for / θ/, /ð/, and /h/. The [+ strident] sounds are: /tʃ/, /dʒ/, /f/, /v/, /s/, /z/, /ʃ/, and /ʒ/.

Labial

The feature of labial refers to place of production. Labial sounds are made with either one or both lips and include bilabials and labio-dentals. The /r/ sound is also considered to have a lip component. The [+ labial] sounds are: /m/, /w/, /p/, /b/, /f/, /v/, and /r/.

Coronal

Coronal sounds refer to production that raises the tongue blade above the neutral state. Typically, these sounds are made with the tongue blade or tongue tip (apex). Sounds with the [+ coronal] feature include: / θ/, /ð/, /s/, /z/, /t/, /d/, /l/, /n/, /ʃ/, /ʒ/, /ʧ/, /ʤ/, /j/, and /r/.

Back

The feature of back refers to a place of production in the velar area that has the tongue body retracted. The [+ back] sounds are: /k/, /g/, /ŋ/, /w/. Of these, the /w/ appears out of place, as it is typically associated with bilabial place. However, in production of the /w/ sound there is a velar component. The most accurate place description for the /w/ is as a labio-velar; however, in working with this sound, speech–language pathologists typically focus on the labial aspect.

Practice in recognizing features is provided in Exercises 39 and 40.

EXERCISE 39

DIRECTIONS: For the following, place a + or − to indicate the value of the feature associated with the phoneme. Keep in mind the basic place, manner, and voicing information associated with each phoneme. That information plus the definitions for the features should help in determining the feature values.

Distinctive Feature	p	b	t	d	k	g	ʧ	ʤ	f	v	θ	ð	s	z	ʃ	ʒ
Sonorant																
Obstruent																
Continuant																
Voice																
Nasal																
Strident																
Labial																
Coronal																
Back																

EXERCISE 40

DIRECTIONS: For the following, place a + or − to indicate the value of the feature associated with the phoneme.

Distinctive Feature	s	z	ʃ	ʒ	h	w	j	l	r	m	n	ŋ
Sonorant												
Obstruent												
Continuant												
Voice												
Nasal												
Strident												
Labial												
Coronal												
Back												

Maximal and Minimal Oppositions

Oppositions have been widely used by clinical researchers and speech–language pathologists in treatment of children with articulation/phonological deficits (Gierut, 1989; Weiner, 1981; Winitz, 1975). Opposition or contrast treatment involves having a child distinguish pairs of syllables or words that vary by a single feature (minimal opposition) or by several features (maximal opposition). Both approaches have been shown to successfully facilitate the acquisition of speech sounds. Exercise 41 gives practice in determining the number of feature differences between sound pairs. Sound pairs that differ by only one feature are considered minimal pairs; those that differ by more than one feature are maximal pairs.

Distinctive Features and Phonological Targets

Distinctive feature analysis describes speech sound errors based on distinctive feature properties. Most systems attempt to determine whether there is a consistent or predominant feature error that accounts for most of the misarticulations. The analysis process begins with collecting a speech sample and identifying sound errors by listing the target sound beside its substitution. Features of the target sound are then compared to those of the substitution. If a particular feature occurs several times across errors, it is targeted for intervention. Figure 2 shows a sample layout using standard transcription format (e.g., p/f means that the [p] sound substitutes for the /f/). The circled items indicate areas where the substitution's feature was different from the target sound's feature. These then would be areas that would be targeted for intervention. In our example the child appears to be having difficulty with [+ continuancy] and [+ stridency] the features associated with the target sounds that are in error. Exercise 42 provides practice in completing a distinctive feature analysis.

EXERCISE 41 ◇◇◇

DIRECTIONS: For the following sound pairs, check the features that differentiate the two sounds and indicate the number of feature differences in the column to the right.

Sound Pair	Sonorant	Obstruent	Continuant	Voice	Nasal	Strident	Labial	Coronal	Back	#
EX: /s/-/m/	✓	✓	✓	✓	✓	✓	✓	✓		8
1. /ŋ/-/p/										
2. /t/-/d/										
3. /g/-/f/										
4. /ʃ/-/h/										
5. /θ/-/b/										
6. /j/-/w/										
7. /ʒ/-/m/										
8. /ð/-/k/										
9. /s/-/d/										
10. /n/-/r/										
11. /s/-/θ/										
12. /tʃ/-/ʃ/										

◇◇◇

Sound Pair	Sonorant	Obstruent	Continuant	Voice	Nasal	Strident	Labial	Coronal	Back
t/s	− −	+ +	(− +)	− −	− −	(− +)	− −	+ +	− −
d/z	− −	+ +	(− +)	+ +	− −	(− +)	− −	+ +	− −
t/ʧ	− −	+ +	− −	− −	− −	(− +)	− −	+ +	− −
p/f	− −	+ +	(− +)	− −	− −	(− +)	+ +	− −	− −
b/v	− −	+ +	(− +)	+ +	− −	(− +)	+ +	− −	− −

FIGURE 2. Distinctive feature analysis.

⬦⬦⬦⬦⬦⬦⬦ EXERCISE 42 ⬦⬦⬦⬦⬦⬦⬦⬦⬦⬦⬦⬦⬦⬦⬦⬦⬦⬦⬦⬦⬦⬦⬦⬦⬦⬦⬦⬦⬦⬦⬦⬦⬦

DIRECTIONS: Complete a distinctive feature analysis on the sample below.

Sound Pair	Sonorant	Obstruent	Continuant	Voice	Nasal	Strident	Labial	Coronal	Back
t/ʃ									
d/g									
t/ʧ									
n/ŋ									
t/k									

Process Descriptions and Scoring Procedures of Common Phonology Assessment Instruments

ALPHA Test of Phonology-Revised

Author: Robert J. Lowe
Copyright: 2000
Publisher: ALPHA Speech & Language Resources
             Box 322
             Mifflinville, PA 18631

The *ALPHA Test of Phonology–Revised* (ALPHA–R) was developed to provide the clinician with the option of completing a traditional analysis (sound by word position) and/or a process description of a child's phonological system. If the child has only a few errors, the ALPHA–R can be used to look at substitutions and omissions in the traditional test format. If enough errors occur for the presence of patterns, however, the sample can also be scored for the presence of phonological processes. The ALPHA–R uses a delayed imitation format to elicit 50 target words embedded in short phrases. Pictures are used to help the child remember the target sentence. In the revised version, the sample can be scored for processes that affect consonants and vowels. Procedures and forms are also available for additional consonant and vowel process analysis based on connected speech sampling.

    The ALPHA–R evaluates for 15 processes affecting consonants. These are defined in Table A.1. As the test is administered, the child's productions are transcribed onto the ALPHA–R protocol using whole-word transcription. During analysis these transcriptions are compared to the target words, and checks are placed in the appropriate process columns facing the transcriptions. Some of the columns have shading, indicating that for a particular word, that process

TABLE A.1

Phonological Processes Evaluated by the *ALPHA Test of Phonology–Revised*

Process	Definition
Consonant deletion	Omission of a consonant in the word-initial or -final position *Note: This does not include consonant sequences*
Syllable deletion	Omission of one syllable of a multisyllable word, usually the weak or unstressed syllable
Stridency deletion	Omission of strident consonants or replacement of them with nonstrident consonants
Stopping	Replacement of continuing consonants or affricates with stop consonants
Fronting	Replacement of back consonants and palatal consonants with consonants produced at or in front of the alveolar ridge
Backing	Replacement of mid and front consonants with back consonants
Alveolarization	Replacement of consonants made with the lips or teeth with consonants made at the alveolar ridge
Labialization	Replacement of consonants made with the tongue tip with consonants made with the lips
Affrication	Replacement of a fricative consonant with an affricate consonant
Deaffrication	Replacement of an affricate consonant with a fricative consonant
Voicing change	Substitution resulting in a change of the voicing feature
Gliding	Replacement of a liquid sound with a glide
Vowelization	Replacement of a liquid sound in word-final position with a vowel
Cluster deletion	Omission of one or more consonants in a consonant cluster
Cluster substitution	Replacement of one or more consonants in a cluster with another consonant

is not a possibility. The columns are wide enough to indicate whether the process is associated with an initial- or a final-word position. To aid in scoring, the ALPHA–R includes an identification matrix. The clinician matches a substitution (column) to its target (row) on the matrix. Where column and row meet are a series of numbers that correspond to the potential phonological processes for that sound change.

The ALPHA–R also evaluates for the presence of 10 vowel processes. These are defined in Table A.2. The vowel processes are scored by comparing the features of height, tenseness, and roundness of the produced vowel with its target. A vowel quadrangle is available on the protocol for making tongue height comparisons. For example, if the child produces [u] for the /o/ phoneme, that would be designated vowel raising, as the /u/ is made with a higher tongue position than the /o/.

TABLE A.2

Vowel Processes Evaluated by the *ALPHA Test of Phonology-Revised*

Process	Definition
Vowel backing	Replacement of a vowel with a more posterior vowel
Vowel lowering	Replacement of a vowel with a vowel made with a lower tongue position
Vowel raising	Replacement of a vowel with a vowel made with a higher tongue position
Centralization	Replacement of a vowel by a vowel with a more central tongue position
Vowel unrounding	Replacement of a normally rounded vowel with a nonrounded vowel
Diphthongization	Production of a monophthong vowel as diphthong
Diphthong reduction	Production of a diphthong as a monophthong
Complete vowel harmony	Change in one vowel so that two vowels in a word are the same
Tenseness harmony	Tensing of a lax vowel in the presence of another tense vowel
Height vowel harmony	Replacement of a vowel by another that is closer in production to height of another vowel in the same word

Bankson–Bernthal Test of Phonology

Author:	Nicholas W. Bankson and
	John E. Bernthal
Copyright:	1990
Publisher:	Paradigm Publishing Company
	16 W. Erie Street, Suite 300
	Chicago, IL 60610

The manual of the *Bankson–Bernthal Test of Phonology* (BBTOP) indicates that the test was developed to assess the phonology of preschool and school-age children. A picture-naming task is used to elicit an 80-word sample from a child. The child's productions of the items are recorded using whole-word transcription, which is later analyzed. The analysis includes three components: consonant inventory, phonological process inventory, and word inventory.

Ten phonological processes are evaluated by the test. A phonological process is defined as "a simplification of a sound class in which target sounds are systematically deleted and/or substituted" (p. 16). Definitions of the 10 processes are presented in Table A.3.

Phonological processes are identified on the BBTOP using the Phonological Process Inventory a full-page grid located on the left side of the protocol booklet (see Figure A.1). The

TABLE A.3

Processes Evaluated by the *Bankson–Bernthal Test of Phonology* (BBTOP)

Process	Definition
Assimilation	Replacement of one sound in a word with a sound that is the same as or similar to a second sound consonant harmony occurring elsewhere in the word *Note: The substituted sound assumes some or all of the characteristics of another sound in the word.*
Fronting	Replacement of a velar sound with one produced farther forward in the oral cavity *Note: Typically an alveolar sound replaces a velar sound.*
Final consonant deletion	Deletion of the final consonant of a word
Weak syllable deletion	Deletion of an unstressed syllable in a word *Note: If more than one syllable is deleted in a word, the production is scored as a weak syllable deletion only once.*
Stopping	Substitution of a stop for a fricative or an affricate (and occasionally for a liquid)
Gliding	Substitution of a glide for a liquid sound before a vowel
Cluster simplification	Simplification of a consonant cluster by deleting one of the consonants *Note: One consonant may be replaced by another, the cluster may be omitted entirely, or the cluster may be replaced.* *Note: Other processes may be reflected in the cluster reductions. For example, /tr/ → [tw] would reflect gliding. For the BBTOP only the cluster simplifications are scored. Gliding is evaluated elsewhere in the test.*
Depalatalization	Movement of the place of articulation of a palatal sound from the palate to a position forward in the mouth, typically the alveolar region
Deaffrication	Replacement of an affricate with a fricative *Note: At times this sound change might also result in depalatalization. The BBTOP does not score depalatalization when it involves affricates being replaced by fricatives.*
Vocalization	Use of a vowel in place of a syllabic or postvocalic liquid *Note: In some regional dialects, changes in vocalic "r" are appropriate and not considered errors.*

facing page shows the consonant inventory, along with target words and the whole-word transcriptions of the client's responses. On the Phonological Process Inventory are 10 columns, one for each of the evaluated processes. In each column, possible productions of target words are entered across from the target word located on the right-hand page. For example, across from the target word *cat* are the productions [tæt] and [tæ] in the "Assimilation" column, [tæ] in the "Fronting" column, and [kæ] and [tæ] in the "Final Consonant Deletion" column.

Phonological Process Inventory

Assimilation	Fronting	Final Consonant Deletion	Weak Syllable Deletion	Stopping	Gliding	Cluster Simplification	Depalatal- ization	Deaffri- cation	Vocal- ization
tæt tæ	tæ	kæ tæ							
det tet gek	de det	ge de							
	tʌp tʌ	kʌ tʌ							
	tændi					kæni kædi			
gɔg dɔd	dɔt	dɔ							
		bɛ							
		bo							
dot do		go do							
gʌŋ	dʌn dʌ	gʌ dʌ							
	taʊ								
	kræ					twæb (kwæb) kæb tæb fræb			
tot kok	to tot dot	ko to							
	wædən	wægə							
	tek ket tet	ke							

(continues)

FIGURE A.1. Example of phonological process inventory from the *Bankson–Bernthal Test of Phonology.*

Note. From *Bankson–Bernthal Test of Phonology,* by N. W. Bankson and J. E. Bernthal, 1990, Chicago: Paradigm. Copyright 1990 by Paradigm Publishing. Reprinted with permission.

Assimilation	Fronting	Final Consonant Deletion	Weak Syllable Deletion	Stopping	Gliding	Cluster Simplification	Depalatal-ization	Deaffri-cation	Vocal-ization
		naɪ		naɪp					
		hæ							
		ræbi wæbɪ			(wæbɪt) wæbɪ				
bənun			bwun bun blun		bəwun bəjun bwun				
					(wæmp) jæmp	læ m læ p			
			redo		(wedio)				
					(weŋ)				
	tɛrət tɛwət	kɛrə	kɛr		(kɛwə t) tɛwə t				kɛət
naɪən			laɪn		(waɪən) jaɪən				
		li		lib	(wif) jif				
		bʌ							
		si di		til di siod					sioʊ sio siə
				tɪd			fɪs		
		sʌ		tʌn					
					7	1			

FIGURE A.1. (*continued*)

The clinician simply checks or circles the word matching his or her client's production of the target.

Some productions may qualify as more than one process. In such cases the clinician should score all possible processes. After scoring all of the productions, the clinician can go back and try to determine which processes most accurately reflect the client's use of the sound system. When the sound changes affect different sounds in the same word, both processes are noted. Some particular sound changes, however, might be scored as more than one process. For example, if the word *cat* were produced [tæt], would the /k/ → [t] sound change be fronting or assimilation? The clinician would have to examine the rest of the child's sample to determine the more accurate description. For guidance in this task, the BBTOP provides some explanation using examples of assimilation and fronting.

Clinical Assessment of Articulation and Phonology

Authors:	Wayne Secord
	JoAnn Donohue
Copyright:	2002
Publisher:	Super Duper Publications
	PO Box 24997
	Greenville, SC 29616

The *Clinical Assessment of Articulation and Phonology* (CAAP) is a norm-referenced assessment that looks at both articulation and phonology. The articulation section has two components: consonant inventory and school-age sentences. The consonant inventory uses a naming task in response to colored pictures. Phonological assessment is based either on responses to the pictures from the consonant inventory component or on the phonological probe section of the test. Ten phonological processes are considered in the evaluation (see Table A.4). Each process is listed on the provided record form, along with the plate number and stimulus word with the target sound boldfaced. A decision rule is provided for each set of stimulus words so that the examiner simply judges whether the rule was met in determining the presence of the phonological process. For example, for Final Consonant Deletion, the final consonant for each stimulus word is boldfaced. The decision rule asks, "Is the final consonant deleted?" The examiner evaluates each stimulus word and answers either *yes* or *no* by putting a checkmark in the provided column. The number of stimulus words for each process ranges from 5 to 10. The number of *yes* responses is added for each process and a percentage of occurrence score determined. Additional phonological process checklists are available in Appendices B and C of the CAAP manual.

TABLE A.4

Phonological Processes Evaluated by the *Clinical Assessment of Articulation and Phonology*

Phonological Process	Description
Final consonant deletion	This process occurs when the final consonant of a syllable, word, or cluster is deleted. The entire cluster must be deleted to be counted as a final consonant deletion.
Cluster reduction	In cluster reduction, one or more consonants are deleted from a two- or three-member consonant cluster. If all members of the cluster are deleted, this is scored as a deletion rather than a reduction.
Syllable reduction	A syllable is deleted from a word containing two or more syllables.
Gliding	The replacement of a liquid with a glide. Gliding can occur in clusters as well.
Vocalization	The replacement of a word-final syllabic consonant or postvocalic liquid by a more neutral vowel.
Fronting	A velar or palatal consonant is replaced by sounds in the front of the mouth.
Deaffrication	An affricate is replaced by a fricative.
Stopping	A fricative or affricate is replaced entirely by a stop consonant.
Prevocalic voicing	An initial voiceless consonant becomes partially or completely voiced.
Postvocalic devoicing	A final voiced consonant becomes partially or completely unvoiced.

Diagnostic Evaluation of Articulation and Phonology

Authors: Barbara Dodd, Zhu Hua, Sharon Crosbie, Alison Holm,
and Anne Ozanne
Copyright: 2006
Publisher: Harcourt Assessment, Inc.
19500 Bulverde Road
San Antonio, TX 78259

The *Diagnostic Evaluation of Articulation and Phonology* (DEAP) is an adaptation of the *Diagnostic Evaluation of Articulation and Phonology* (2002), developed in the United Kingdom. The DEAP was designed to provide differential diagnoses between articulation and phonological speech disorders and has been norm-referenced for children in the United States between the ages of 3 years and 8 years 11 months. It differentiates among four speech disorder subgroups: articulation disorders, phonological delay, consistent phonological disorder, and inconsistent phonological disorder. The DEAP includes five tests, two of which are screenings and three of which are assessments. Results of an initial screening test indicate whether further testing is needed and which additional assessment is to be administered.

The Phonology Assessment uses both picture naming and connected speech in evaluating speech-sound production. For the picture naming, the child is asked to label 50 colored pictures. The words are primarily nouns but include one-, two-, three-, and even four-syllable items. If the child does not know the item, the test administrator can provide a forced choice or go to direct imitation. In the connected speech task the examiner asks the child to describe three scenes that depict unusual or funny situations (e.g., a giraffe carrying a picnic basket). Four or five target words are embedded in each picture. These words are also found in the picture naming section of the assessment, which allows for a check on production consistency.

The DEAP identifies 10 common processes but includes a column for "Other Error Patterns." Appendix G of the DEAP manual includes descriptions and examples of the common error patterns and four atypical error patterns. The score form is designed with the target word and transcription on the left and potential error patterns on the right. Common errors are listed under each pattern to help with the identification. Table A.5 lists the error patterns evaluated by the DEAP.

The DEAP includes a separate assessment for evaluating articulation errors. The child is asked to name 30 pictured items, which are scored for consonantal errors in the initial and final positions of syllables. Nineteen vowels are also elicited during this task.

TABLE A.5

Phonological Patterns Evaluated by the *Diagnostic Evaluation of Articulation and Phonology*

Pattern	Definition
Gliding	A liquid, nasal, or stop consonant is replaced with a glide.
Vocalization of liquids	A liquid (/ɚ/ or /l/) occurring after a vowel is replaced with a vowel.
Deaffrication	An affricate is replaced with a fricative.
Cluster reduction	One or more consonants are deleted from a cluster.
Fronting	The target consonant's place of articulation is moved to a more anterior position.
Weak syllable deletion	An unstressed syllable is deleted.
Stopping	A consonant, typically a fricative or affricate, is replaced with a stop consonant. Other consonants (glides, liquids, nasals) may also be replaced with stop consonants.
Prevocalic voicing	A voiceless consonant is replaced with a voiced consonant.
Postvocalic devoicing	A final voiced consonant is replaced with a voiceless consonant.
Final consonant deletion	A consonant is deleted at the end of a syllable. If a cluster appears at the end of the syllable, all of the cluster members must be deleted.

Hodson Assessment of Phonological Patterns–Third Edition

Author: Barbara Williams Hodson
Copyright: 2004
Publisher: PRO-ED, Inc.
              8700 Shoal Creek Blvd.
              Austin, TX 78757-6897

The *Hodson Assessment of Phonological Patterns–Third Edition* (HAPP-3) is the latest version of the *Assessment of Phonological Processes–Revised* (APP-R). It was designed to assess phonological deviations found in children with highly unintelligible speech. This latest version of the test updates and internationalizes the target words and transcriptions, provides more user-friendly forms, includes the objects to be used in eliciting the targets words, and provides normative scores.

As in the previous edition, the HAPP-3 uses stimulus objects and pictures to elicit 50 stimulus words through a naming task. The target words are transcribed onto Section 10 of the Record Form. The information from Section 10 is transferred to the Major Phonological Deviations Analysis Form, where the sound changes are coded as either word/syllable structures (omissions) or consonant category deficiencies. The manual provides details for scoring the sound changes. The Substitutions and Other Strategies Analysis Form is used to record substitutions, distortions, additions, and position changes in a word (see Table A.6). The information is summarized on the Major Phonological Deviations Analysis Form. Ability (standard score) scores and percentile ranks are available for ages 3 years through 7 years 11 months.

The HAPP-3 also includes two screening instruments. The Preschool Phonological Screening Instrument examines consonant omissions and substitutions based on 12 target words. The Multisyllabic Word Screening Instrument looks at speech production in 12 polysyllabic words or two-word phrases. This screening looks for consonant omissions, metathesis, and various assimilations.

Khan-Lewis Phonological Analysis–Second Edition

Author: Linda M. L. Khan and Nancy P. Lewis
Copyright: 2002
Publisher: American Guidance Service, Inc.
              4201 Woodlane Road
              Circle Pines, MN 55041-1796

The *Khan-Lewis Phonological Analysis–Second Edition* (KLPA-2) is the second edition of the *Khan-Lewis Phonological Analysis*, first published in 1986. The KLPA-2 is designed to be used as a supplement to the *Goldman-Fristoe Test of Articulation–Second Edition* (GFTA-2). The

TABLE A.6

Substitutions and Other Strategies From the *Hodson Assessment
of Phonological Patterns–Third Edition*

Substitutions and other strategies	Description
Glottal Stop replacement	Production of a glottal stop in place of another phoneme.
Stopping	Substitution of a stop consonant for a continuant (fricative, liquid, glide) phoneme.
Fronting	Substitution of an anterior consonant for a posterior consonant.
Backing	Substitution of a posterior consonant for an anterior consonant.
Gliding	Substitution of glides /w/ and /j/ for other phonemes.
Vowelization	Substitution of a vowel for a consonant.
Metathesis	Transposition of phonemes or syllables. Can occur across word boundaries as well as within words.
Migration	Similar to metathesis; however, only one phoneme is moved to another place in a word.
Affrication	Addition of a stop component to a continuant phoneme.
Deaffrication	Changing an affricate target phoneme to a continuant or a stop.
Palatalization	Addition of a palatal component to a nonpalatal target phoneme.
Depalatalization	Deletion of a palatal component from a palatal target phoneme.
Labial assimilation	A nonlabial target becomes labial because of another labial consonant in the context.
Nasal assimilation	A nonnasal target becomes nasal because of another nasal consonant in the context.
Velar assimilation	A velar is substituted for a nonvelar consonant because of another velar in the word context.
Other assimilations	A sound change occurs due to the influence of another sound in the word context.
Coalescence	Replacement of two phonemes by a new phoneme that has characteristics of both the original phonemes.
Reduplication	Repetition of phonemes or syllables.
Vowel deviations	Production of phonemic vowel substitutions that affect meaning. Allophone variations, minimal vowel alterations, dialectal variations not included.
Prevocalic voicing	A voiceless prevocalic consonant is replaced by a voiced consonant.
Prevocalic devoicing	A prevocalic voiced consonant is replaced by a voiceless consonant.
Postvocalic devoicing	A postvocalic voiced consonant is replaced by a voiceless consonant.
Epenthesis	A vowel is inserted, typically between members of a cluster.

KLPA-2 assesses the use of 10 phonological processes as determined by responses to the 53 target words elicited from the Sounds-in-Words section of the GFTA-2. See Table A.7 for descriptions of the 10 phonological processes.

The KLPA-2 provides standard scores, confidence intervals, and percentiles for ages 2 through 21 years 11 months based on a large, nationally representative reference group. In addition to the 10 targeted phonological processes, the authors of the KLPA-2 encourage the assessment of 34 other phonological processes and vowel alterations. Detailed descriptions of the various processes are available in the manual. To facilitate identification of processes, a sound-change booklet is also provided. This booklet takes each target word from the GFTA-2 and matches up potential sound changes with phonological processes. The booklet is color coded following the initial, medial, and final position coding found in the GFTA-2.

The KLPA-2 scoring form has been simplified from the original version. Target words and transcriptions are presented on the left side of the form with room to enter information from the GFTA-2. In the middle of the form, the 10 phonological processes are arranged in columns. There is space for noting additional processes and vowel alterations in columns on the right side. Using the Sound Change Booklet, the test administrator can place check marks across from the target word and under the name of the identified phonological processes. Processes that are not applicable to target words are blocked out in blue. Based on the total raw score, the normative tables can then be used to derive a standard score, confidence interval, percentile, and test-age equivalent.

Smit–Hand Articulation and Phonology Evaluation

Author:	Ann Bosma Smit and Linda Hand
Copyright:	1997
Publisher:	Western Psychological Services
	12031 Wilshire Boulevard
	Los Angeles, CA 90025-1251

The *Smit–Hand Articulation and Phonology Evaluation* (SHAPE) was developed to provide both an independent (speech system viewed as self-contained) and a relational (child system compared with adult system) analysis. The assessment provides normative data for children between 3 and 9 years of age. The SHAPE relies on 80 color photographs to elicit 108 target speech productions. There are multiple exemplars of several of the phonemes and clusters. Productions are elicited through spontaneous naming of the pictures. Sentences are provided that help provide cues to the child about categories of pictured objects that will be shown. Some pictures have cue sentences to facilitate elicitation of the target word. If the child does not respond correctly, the clinician provides a forced choice option ("Is it [target] or [alternative]?"); if that fails, the clinician provides a direct model to be imitated. The "Record Booklet" provides boxes that can be checked to indicate if direct or delayed imitation was needed in eliciting the target.

TABLE A.7

Developmental Processes Evaluated by the *Khan-Lewis Phonological Analysis–Second Edition*

Process	Definition
Deletion of final consonants	Deletion or the final consonant of final cluster of a word
Initial voicing	Use of voiced consonants to begin words that should begin with voiceless consonants *Note: Place and manner of articulation may or may not be altered.*
Syllable reduction	Reduction in the number of syllables in the target word
Palatal fronting	Fronting of a palatal consonant, usually to the alveolar ridge
Deaffrication	Deletion of the stop feature of an affricate, with retention of fricative or continuant feature *Note: Deaffrication may interact with palatal fronting.*
Velar fronting	Production of an alveolar consonant for a target velar consonant in a syllable or word
Stopping of fricatives and affricates	Stopping of a fricative, resulting in affricates or stops; or stopping of affricates, resulting in stop consonants *Note: Stopping of glides or nasals is not included in this category.*
Cluster simplification	Simplification of a consonant sequence (cluster) by deleting one or more of the consonants or by inserting a schwa vowel between them
Final devoicing	Deletion of voicing in word-final voiced consonants, leading to production as voiceless consonants
Liquid simplification	Gliding or vocalization of liquids
Gliding of liquids	Production of liquids (/l/ and /r/) as glides (/w/ and /j/)
Vocalization of liquids	Production of a vowel for the syllabics /l/ and /r/

A unique feature of the SHAPE is its scoring and analysis. A "Record Booklet" is used for collecting the elicited speech sample. Each target word is listed with the target sounds in bold face. Below the target word is a row of boxes containing the correct production and several common errors associated with the target sound. The clinician simply circles the number above the box containing the target or the error the child has made. Another unique feature of the SHAPE is its use of "Verbal Descriptors." Various descriptors (e.g., dentalized, partially devoiced, labialized) are listed with different targets and can be checked to provide a more detailed description of how the target sound was articulated. The information from the record booklet is transferred to an extensive "AutoScore Form" (12 pages), which is used for analysis. The "AutoScore Form" uses carbon paper to register information into different areas to facilitate the analysis. The analysis includes: Phonetic Inventory, Syllable Inventory, Word Shape Inventory, Contrast Analysis, Common Phonological Processes, and Idiosyncratic Processes.

The SHAPE identifies 11 common phonological processes through its formal scoring system (Table A.8). The instrument also provides information for determining whether a given process meets a 40% use criterion and, if so, means for determining the exact percentage of use. Another nine processes considered rare (idiosyncratic) are defined in the manual's appendix (see Table A.9).

TABLE A.8

Phonological Processes Evaluated by the *Smit–Hand Articulation and Phonology Evaluation*

Process	Definition
Final consonant deletion	Deletion of a targeted final consonant obstruent singleton
Cluster reduction /s/ clusters	Deletion of one or more of the consonant members in /s/ clusters
Cluster reduction /l/, /r/, /w/ cluster	Deletion of one or more of the consonant members in /l/, /r/, or /w/ clusters
Weak syllable deletion	Deletion of one or more syllables of a polysyllabic word
Voicing of initial voiceless consonants	Replacement of initial singleton consonants that are phonemically (originally) voiceless by a voiced consonant
Stopping of initial fricatives and affricate singles	Use of a stop for an initial fricative or affricate
Fronting of initial velar singletons	Use of an alveolar for a target velar
Depalatalization of initial singletons	Replacement of an initial palatal singleton with a more anterior consonant
Depalatalization of final singletons	Replacement of a final palatal singleton with a more anterior consonant
Gliding of initial liquids	Replacement of initial /l/ or /r/ with /h/, /w/ or /j/
Vocalization of final and postvocalic liquids	Replacement of final /l/ or /r/ by a vowel

TABLE A.9

Idiosyncratic Processes Defined by *Smit–Hand Articulation and Phonology Evaluation*

Process	Definition
Deletion of initial consonants	Deletion of singleton consonants in word-initial position
Glottal substitution for initial obstruents	Replacement of word-initial singleton obstruents (with exception of /t/) with a glottal stop
Glottal substitution for final obstruents	Replacement of final singleton obstruents (with exception of /t/) with a glottal stop
Stopping of final fricatives and affricates	Replacement of final singleton fricatives or affricates with a stop
Stopping of fricatives in clusters	Replacement of the fricative in a cluster with a stop
Backing of initial alveolar consonants	Replacement of an alveolar singleton consonant in word-initial position with a velar consonant
Backing of final alveolar consonants	Replacement of an alveolar singleton consonant in word-final position with a velar consonant
Epenthesis	The addition of a consonant, a vowel, or one or more syllables to a target word *Note: Insertion of the schwa vowel in a cluster is not considered an error.*
Assimilation processes	Alteration of one consonant in a word to become more like another consonant elsewhere in the word *Note: The following assimilation processes are considered:* regressive labial assimilation regressive alveolar assimilation (affecting stops) regressive velar assimilation (affecting alveolars) regressive nasal assimilation progressive labial assimilation progressive alveolar assimilation (affecting velars) progressive velar assimilation (affecting alveolars and palatals)

Structured Photographic Articulation Test II: Featuring Dudsberry

Author:	Janet I. Dawson and Patricia J. Tattersall
Copyright:	2001
Publisher:	Janelle Publications
	PO Box 811
	1189 Twombley Road
	DeKalb, IL 60115

The *Structured Photographic Articulation Test II: Featuring Dudsberry* (SPAT-D II) utilizes 40 photographs featuring a golden retriever named Dudsberry to elicit sounds at the word level for analysis of articulation and phonological processes. As the photographs are shown, the child is asked to name the picture or finish a phrase related to the photograph started by the clinician. An additional eight photographs are used to elicit sounds in connected speech, either as a sentence imitation task or, if the child is old enough, through reading.

The SPAT-D II evaluates nine phonological processes (see Table A.10). There are several opportunities for each process. The manual provides a breakdown of words and potential processes by initial, medial, and final word position. A percentage of occurrence for each process is calculated by dividing the number of occurrences by the number of opportunities of occurrence (found on score sheet). Appendix D provides a Phonological Process Identification Chart to help identify processes associated with sound changes. The chart is laid out as a matrix with potential substitutions across the top and target phonemes down the left side. Processes are identified at the intersection of target phoneme and substitution on the matrix by use of process abbreviations with a key at the bottom of the chart. Normative data are provided for the articulation component of the assessment but not for the phonological processes.

TABLE A.10

Phonological Processes Identified by the *Structured Photographic Articulation Test II: Featuring Dudsberry*

Process	Definition
Initial consonant deletion	The omission of the initial consonant sound.
Final consonant deletion	Omission of the final consonant of a word.
Stridency deletion	Omission of a strident consonant or replacement of a strident consonant by a nonstrident consonant.
Stopping	Replacement of a fricative or affricate with a stop consonant.
Palatal fronting	Replacement of a palatal fricative or affricate with a more anterior consonant.
Velar fronting	Replacement of a velar consonant with a consonant made anterior to the palatal place of articulation.
Gliding of liquids	Replacement of an initial or medial liquid with a glide.
Cluster reduction	The omission of one or more consonants in a cluster comprising two or more consonants.
Syllable reduction	The omission of one or more syllables of a multisyllabic word.

Answers to Exercises
and Mini-Quizzes

EXERCISE 1 ◇◇

Characteristics	Speech Sound
1. Voiced, lingua-alveolar, plosive	/d/
2. Voiceless, lingua-dental, fricative	/θ/
3. Voiced, palatal, glide	/j/
4. Voiced, labio-dental, fricative	/v/
5. Voiced, velar, nasal	/ŋ/
6. Voiced, palatal, fricative	/ʒ/
7. Voiceless, lingua-alveolar, plosive	/t/
8. Voiceless, palatal, affricate	/ʧ/
9. Voiced, lingua-alveolar, liquid	/l/
10. Voiced, velar, plosive	/g/

EXERCISE 2 ◇◇

Sound	Voicing	Place	Manner
1. /w/	voiced	bilabial	glide
2. /z/	voiced	lingua-alveolar	fricative
3. /h/	voiceless	glottal	fricative
4. /b/	voiced	bilabial	stop-plosive
5. /f/	voiceless	labio-dental	fricative
6. /ʃ/	voiceless	palatal	fricative
7. /n/	voiced	lingua-alveolar	nasal
8. /ʤ/	voiced	palatal	affricate
9. /k/	voiceless	velar	stop-plosive
10. /r/	voiced	palatal	liquid

EXERCISE 3

Group	Sounds
1. All voiced labials	/ b /, / v /, / m /, / w /
2. All voiced fricatives	/ ʒ /, / z /, / ð /, / v /
3. All velars	/ k /, / g /, / ŋ /
4. All palatals	/r /, / j /, / ʃ /, / ʒ /, / tʃ /, / dʒ /
5. All nonstrident fricatives	/h/, / θ /, / ð /
6. All strident lingual fricatives	/ ʃ /, / ʒ /, / s /, / z /
7. All strident nonfricatives	/ tʃ /, / dʒ /
8. All strident obstruents	/ tʃ /, / dʒ /, / ʃ /, / ʒ /, /s /, / z /, / f /, / v /
9. All voiceless, labial obstruents	/ f /, / p /
10. All palatal fricatives	/ ʃ /, / ʒ /

EXERCISE 4

Sounds	Group
1. /v/, /b/, /m/	all voiced labials
2. /d/, /n/, /s/, /z/	all alveolar
3. /h/, /θ/, /ð/	all nonstrident fricatives
4. /b/, /g/, /d/	all voiced stop-plosives
5. /j/, /r/, /ʃ/, /tʃ/, /dʒ/, /ʒ/	all palatal sounds
6. /tʃ/, /t/, /s/, /k/, /p/	all voiceless (all obstruents)
7. /k/, /g/, /ŋ/	all velars
8. /z/, /ʒ/, /v/, /ð/	all voiced fricatives
9. /ʃ/, /tʃ/	all voiceless palatals
10. /θ/, /s/, /ʃ/, /f/	all voiceless fricatives

EXERCISE 5 ◇◇◇

Features	Vowel
1. High-mid, front	/ ɪ /
2. Low-mid, back	/ ɔ /
3. Mid, front	/ e /
4. Low-mid, front	/ ɛ /
5. Low-mid, central	/ ʌ /
6. High-mid, back	/ ʊ /
7. Low, back	/ ɑ /
8. Mid-central, tense, rounded	/ ɝ /
9. Mid-back	/ o /
10. Low, front	/ æ /

EXERCISE 6 ◇◇◇

Front	Central	Back	
/i/		/u/	High
/ɪ/		/ʊ/	High-mid
/e/	/ ɝ / / ə / / ɚ /	/o/	Mid
/ɛ/	/ ʌ /	/ɔ/	Low-mid
/æ/		/ɑ/	Low

◇◇

EXERCISE 7

Word	Diphthong
1. joy	/ ɔɪ /
2. how	/ aʊ /
3. air	/ ɛr /
4. show	/ oʊ /
5. high	/ aɪ /
6. now	/ aʊ /
7. rode	/ oʊ /
8. Roy	/ ɔɪ /
9. mine	/ aɪ /
10. save	/ eɪ /
11. car	/ ɑr /
12. store	/ ɔr /
13. made	/ eɪ /
14. beer	/ ɪr /

EXERCISE 8 ◇◇

| Target Word | | Processes | | | | | |
	Syllable Deletion	Reduplication	Epenthesis	Final-Consonant Deletion	Initial-Consonant Deletion	Cluster Deletion	Cluster Substitution
Ex: *boat*				✓	✓		
1. bed				✓	✓		
2. goat				✓	✓		
3. grape			✓	✓		✓	✓
4. bucket	✓	✓		✓	✓		
5. nest			✓		✓	✓	✓
6. mouse				✓	✓		
7. tribe			✓	✓		✓	✓
8. cry			✓			✓	✓
9. stone			✓	✓		✓	✓
10. ouch				✓			
11. tomato	✓	✓			✓		
12. tan				✓	✓		
13. east			✓			✓	✓
14. stray			✓			✓	✓
15. trapper	✓	✓	✓			✓	✓

◇◇◇

EXERCISE 9

Target	Initial-Consonant Deletion	Final-Consonant Deletion	Cluster Deletion
Ex: *stoop*	NA	[stu]	[tup] or [sup] or [up]
1. taste	[est]	NA	[tet] or [tes] or [te]
2. seed	[id]	[si]	NA
3. steep	NA	[sti]	[tip] or [sip] or [ip]
4. slip	NA	[slɪ]	[lɪp] or [sɪp] or [ɪp]
5. bread	NA	[brɛ]	[bɛd] or [rɛd] or [ɛd]
6. road	[od]	[ro]	NA
7. park	[ɑrk]	[pɑr]	NA
8. plate	NA	[ple]	[pet] or [let] or [et]
9. mash	[æʃ]	[mæ]	NA
10. brave	NA	[bre]	[bev] or [rev] or [ev]

EXERCISE 10

Target	Child Form	Answer
1. blue	[bu]	partial
2. beast	[bi]	total
3. glue	[gwu]	substitution
4. spoon	[pun]	partial
5. tree	[twi]	substitution
6. claw	[kɪ]	partial
7. skate	[eɪ]	total
8. slow	[wo]	partial and substitution
9. plate	[pweɪt]	substitution
10. straight	[tweɪt]	partial and substitution

EXERCISE 11

Target	Total Cluster Deletion	Partial Cluster Deletion	Cluster Substitution
1. play	[eɪ]	[peɪ]	[pweɪ]
2. clay	[eɪ]	[keɪ]	[kweɪ]
3. sleep	[ip]	[lip]	[swip]
4. break	[eɪk]	[beɪk]	[bweɪk]
5. block	[ɔk]	[bɔk]	[bwɔk]
6. strong	[ɔŋ]	[trɔŋ]	[stwɔŋ]
7. prom	[ɔm]	[pɔm]	[pwɔm]
8. creek	[ik]	[kik]	[kwik]
9. grape	[eɪp]	[geɪp]	[gweɪp]
10. string	[ɪŋ]	[trɪŋ]	[stwɪŋ]

Note. It is typically the more difficult sounds that are deleted or substituted.

EXERCISE 12

Target	Child Form	Answer
1. water	[wɑwɑ]	Total
2. blanket	[didi]	Total
3. bottle	[bɑdɑ]	Partial
4. daddy	[dædɑ]	Partial
5. candy	[kɑki]	Partial
6. pillow	[pɑpo]	Partial
7. puppy	[pɑpɑ]	Total
8. nanny	[nɑnɑ]	Total
9. bottle	[bɑbi]	Partial
10. baby	[beɪbe]	Total

EXERCISE 13

Target	Answer
1. space	[səpeɪs]
2. train	[təreɪn]
3. play	[pəleɪ]
4. black	[bəlæk]
5. steak	[səteɪk]

EXERCISE 14 ◇◇

NOTES: More than one sound change can occur in a target word. In #3 below, the word *grape* has a change in the word-initial cluster and in the final consonant. Always examine the entire word when assessing for sound changes.

Sometimes the major change is in the number of syllables, as in #11.

For reduplication, the clinician must be alert for repeating syllables that do not match up to the target word syllables. In #4, bucket, the second syllable of the child form is not even close to that of the target word, but it is similar to the first syllable.

						Processes			
Target	**Child Form**	**Sound Change**	Syllable Deletion	Reduplication	Epenthesis	Final-Consonant Deletion	Initial-Consonant Deletion	Cluster Deletion	Cluster Substitution
Ex: *boat*	[bo]	t → ∅				✓			
1. bed	[ɛd]	b → ∅					✓		
2. goat	[o]	g → ∅ t → ∅				✓	✓		
3. grape	[gəreɪ]	gr → gər			✓	✓			
4. bucket	[bʌbɑ]	cvcvc → cvcv	✓			✓			
5. nest	[nɛt]	st → t						✓	
6. mouse	[maʊ]	s → ∅				✓			
7. tribe	[twaɪ]	tr → tw b → ∅				✓			✓
8. cry	[kaɪ]	kr → k						✓	
9. stone	[on]	st → ∅						✓	
10. ouch	[aʊ]	tʃ → ∅				✓			
11. tomato	[meɪdo]	cvcvcv → cvcv	✓						
12. tan	[{n]	t → ∅					✓		
13. east	[it]	st → t						✓	
14. stray	[tweɪ]	str → tw						✓	✓
15. trapper	[təræpə]	tr → tər ɚ → ə			✓				

◇◇

◇◇◇◇◇◇◇◇ **EXERCISE 15** ◇◇◇

NOTES: Remember, the fricatives and affricates are strident except for /h/, /θ/, and /ð/

Stopping can affect all of the sounds.

Target	Child Form	Process
Ex: save	[teɪv]	stopping, stridency deletion
1. soup	[tup]	stopping, stridency deletion
2. thin	[tɪn]	stopping
3. base	[beɪt]	stopping, stridency deletion
4. house	[taʊf]	stopping
5. moose	[mut]	stopping, stridency deletion
6. feet	[tit]	stopping, stridency deletion
7. zoo	[du]	stopping, stridency deletion
8. chase	[teɪs]	stopping, stridency deletion
9. shake	[teɪk]	stopping, stridency deletion
10. bath	[bæt]	stopping

◇◇◇

EXERCISE 16 ◇◇

NOTES: Since the instructions are to mark all *possible* processes, some unlikely sound changes will still be scored. A good example is #2, *think*, it is unlikely that the /θ/ would be produced as an affricate, but it is possible, since the /θ/is a fricative.

Number 13, *ghost*, has an /st/ cluster. Clusters are scored as separate entities, and thus those sounds should not be considered here for processes such as stopping, fronting, and affrication.

Target Word	Stopping	Stridency Deletion	Fronting	Depalatalization	Palatalization	Affrication	Deaffrication
				Process			
Ex: *suit*	✓	✓			✓	✓	
1. judge	✓	✓	✓	✓			✓
2. think	✓				✓	✓	
3. kiss	✓	✓	✓		✓	✓	
4. cheese	✓	✓	✓	✓	✓	✓	✓
5. sun	✓	✓			✓	✓	
6. moose	✓	✓			✓	✓	
7. case	✓	✓	✓		✓	✓	
8. math	✓				✓	✓	
9. shirt	✓	✓	✓	✓	✓	✓	
10. page	✓	✓	✓	✓	✓		✓
11. path	✓				✓	✓	
12. zoo	✓	✓			✓	✓	
13. ghost			✓		✓		
14. John	✓	✓	✓	✓			✓
15. face	✓	✓			✓	✓	

◇◇

◇◇◇◇◇◇◇◇ **EXERCISE 17** ◇◇◇◇◇◇◇◇◇◇◇◇◇◇◇◇◇◇◇◇◇◇◇◇◇◇◇◇◇◇◇◇◇◇◇◇◇◇

NOTES: As in previous exercises, the first step is to identify the sound changes. Many times the changes occur in both initial- and word-final positions. Remember that clusters are not scored for any processes except cluster substitution and deletion. Thus, the /ŋk/ to [nt] changes in the word *think* could be scored as cluster substitution but not as fronting. Similarly the /st/ in *ghost* could be scored only under cluster deletion.

Target	Child Form	Sound Change	Stopping	Stridency Deletion	Fronting	Depalatalization	Palatalization	Affrication	Deaffrication
Ex: *suit*	[tut]	s → t	✓	✓			✓	✓	
1. judge	[dʌd]	ʤ → d ʤ → d	✓	✓	✓	✓			✓
2. think	[tɪnt]	θ → t ŋ → nt	✓						
3. kiss	[tɪt]	k → t s → t	✓	✓	✓				
4. cheese	[tid]	ʧ → t z → d	✓	✓	✓	✓			✓
5. sun	[ʃʌn]	s → ʃ					✓		
6. moose	[muʧ]	s → ʧ					✓	✓	
7. case	[teʃ]	k → t s → ʃ			✓		✓		
8. math	[mæʧ]	θ → ʧ					✓	✓	
9. shirt	[sɝt]	ʃ → s			✓	✓			
10. page	[ped]	ʤ → d	✓	✓	✓	✓			✓
11. path	[pæt]	θ → t	✓						
12. zoo	[ʤu]	z → ʤ					✓	✓	
13. ghost	[dot]	g → d			✓				
14. John	[dɑn]	ʤ → d	✓	✓	✓	✓			✓
15. face	[peʧ]	f → p s → ʧ	✓	✓			✓	✓	

EXERCISE 18

NOTE: In most cases the / l / in the word *limb* (#12) would change to a [w] and be labeled gliding.

	Process				
Target Word	**Backing**	**Gliding**	**Alveolarization**	**Labialization**	**Vowelization**
Ex: *suit*	✓			✓	
1. cave	✓		✓		
2. lake		✓			
3. take	✓			✓	
4. ram	✓	✓	✓		
5. shoe	✓				
6. beetle	✓		✓		✓
7. face	✓		✓	✓	
8. math	✓		✓	✓	
9. button	✓		✓	✓	✓
10. pace	✓		✓	✓	
11. bath	✓		✓	✓	
12. limb	✓	✓	✓		
13. goat	✓			✓	
14. job	✓		✓		
15. rode	✓	✓		✓	

◇◇◇◇◇◇◇◇ **EXERCISE 19** ◇◇◇◇◇◇◇◇◇◇◇◇◇◇◇◇◇◇◇◇◇◇◇◇◇◇◇◇◇◇◇◇◇◇◇

Target	Child Form	Sound Change	Backing	Gliding	Alveolarization	Labialization	Vowelization
Ex: *suit*	[kut]	s → k	✓				
1. cave	[ted]	k → t v → d			✓		
2. lake	[wek]	l → w		✓			
3. take	[kek]	t → k	✓				
4. ram	[jæm]	r → j		✓			
5. shoe	[ku]	ʃ → k	✓				
6. beetle	[bido]	l → o					✓
7. face	[fef]	s → f				✓	
8. math	[mæf]	θ → f				✓	
9. button	[bʌtɑ]	n → ɑ					✓
10. pace	[kef]	p → k s → f	✓			✓	
11. bath	[bæt]	θ → t			✓		
12. limb	[wɪm]	l → w		✓			
13. goat	[gok]	t → k	✓				
14. job	[gɔd]	ʤ → g b → d	✓		✓		
15. rode	[wog]	r → w d → g	✓	✓			

◇◇◇

EXERCISE 20

Target	Child Form	Sound Change	Backing	Fronting	Stopping	Stridency Deletion	Deaffrication	Depalatalization	Gliding	Affrication	Labialization
							Process				
Ex: seed	[tid]	s → t			✓	✓					
1. sheet	[it]	ʃ → ø				✓					
2. gate	[det]	g → d		✓							
3. chase	[tef]	tʃ → t s → f		✓	✓	✓	✓	✓			✓
4. lady	[wedɪ]	l → w							✓		
5. page	[pedz]	dʒ → dz		✓				✓			
6. moth	[mɔf]	θ → f									✓
7. reef	[wip]	r → w f → p			✓	✓			✓		
8. same	[kem]	s → k	✓		✓	✓					
9. nose	[nod]	z → d			✓	✓					
10. booth	[buf]	θ → f									✓
11. mice	[naɪtʃ]	m → n s → tʃ								✓	
12. choke	[tot]	tʃ → t k → t		✓	✓	✓	✓	✓			
13. Joe	[go]	dʒ → g	✓		✓	✓	✓	✓			
14. leash	[wis]	l → w ʃ → s			✓				✓	✓	
15. gas	[dæt]	g → d s → t		✓	✓	✓					

◇◇◇◇◇◇◇◇◇ MINI-QUIZ 1 ◇◇◇

a. reduplication
b. initial-consonant deletion
c. stopping
d. backing
e. labialization
f. partial
g. obstruents
h. deaffrication
i. gliding

j. fronting
k. weak
l. stridency deletion
m. final-consonant deletion
n. alveolarization
o. cluster deletion
p. labial
q. sonorants
r. palatalization

1. __j__ process by which velars and palatals are replaced by alveolars
2. __f__ type of reduplication that occurs when the two syllables are not identical
3. __l__ process suggested by the deletion of an /s/, regardless of word position
4. __n__ process by which labials or interdentals are replaced by alveolar sounds
5. __i__ process that affects both of the liquids
6. __o__ EX: /stov/ becoming [tov]
7. __r__ process suggested by the replacement of an /s/ with a /ʃ/
8. __q__ group that includes nasals, glides, and liquids
9. __k__ syllable typically deleted in syllable deletion
10. __h__ process suggested by the replacement of /tʃ/ with /s/
11. __g__ category made up of the fricatives, affricates, and stops
12. __b__ EX: /bot/ changing to [ot]
13. __d__ EX: /to/ changing to [ko]
14. __p__ place in which /w/, /p/, and /f/ are produced

EXERCISE 21 ◇◇

NOTES: To determine whether an assimilation is regressive or progressive, you must look at the relationship between the sound that changed and the sound that influenced the change. If the sound that changed occurs first, the assimilation is regressive. If it occurs after the influencing sound, the assimilation is progressive.

Contiguity is determined by the presence or absence of intervening segments between the sound that changes and its influencing sound.

Target	Child Form	Answer
Ex: *soap*	[pop]	regressive, noncontiguous
1. coat	[tot]	regressive, noncontiguous
2. take	[teɪt]	progressive, noncontiguous
3. suit	[zut]	regressive, contiguous (voicing of vowel)
4. cat	[kæk]	progressive, noncontiguous
5. sheet	[sit]	regressive, noncontiguous
6. face	[feɪf]	progressive, noncontiguous
7. room	[wum]	regressive, noncontiguous
8. shake	[keɪk]	regressive, noncontiguous
9. break	[bweɪk]	progressive, contiguous
10. tack	[tæt]	progressive, noncontiguous
11. goat	[gok]	progressive, noncontiguous
12. lame	[weɪm]	regressive, noncontiguous
13. sad	[tæd]	regressive, noncontiguous
14. safe	[feɪf]	regressive, noncontiguous
15. thumb	[fʌm]	regressive, noncontiguous

◇◇

EXERCISE 22

NOTE: In assimilation, a sound changes to become more like another sound in the same phonetic environment. After you identify a sound change, try to determine if the sound has become more like another sound in the same word.

If so, then the sound change may be due to assimilation.

Target Word	Child Form	Sound Change	Assimilation Maybe	No
Ex: co*a*t	[tot]	k → t	X	
co*a*t	[kod]	t → d		X
1. take	[teɪt]	k → t	X	
2. lame	[deɪm]	l → d		X
3. sheet	[tit]	ʃ → t	X	
4. tape	[keɪp]	t → k		X
5. tip	[kɪp]	t → k		X
6. case	[seɪs]	k → s	X	
7. tack	[tæg]	k → g		X
8. shake	[geɪk]	ʃ → g	X	
9. face	[veɪs]	f → v	X	
10. leaf	[wif]	l → w	X	

EXERCISE 23

NOTE: For prevocalic voicing to occur, the target word must begin with a voiceless consonant.

<u>shoe</u>	bad	<u>patch</u>
<u>cake</u>	<u>thumb</u>	<u>kitty</u>
got	<u>coat</u>	bye-bye
<u>chips</u>	run	<u>candy</u>
<u>sock</u>	<u>fun</u>	that

EXERCISE 24 ◇◇

NOTE: For postvocalic devoicing to occur, the target word must end with a voiced consonant.

this	<u>pad</u>	pitch
<u>nose</u>	<u>save</u>	half
<u>rub</u>	cot	leash
<u>lid</u>	bike	<u>have</u>
<u>judge</u>	<u>kid</u>	<u>rose</u>

EXERCISE 25 ◇◇

Target Word	Child Form	Sound Change	PrV	PDe	Neither
Ex: *tape*	[deɪp]	t → d	X		
1. robe	[rop]	b → p		X	
2. two	[du]	t → d	X		
3. seed	[dit]	s → d d → t	X	X	
4. made	[meɪt]	d → t		X	
5. sad	[tæd]	s → t			X
6. page	[peɪs]	ʤ → s		X	
7. Sue	[du]	s → d	X		
8. nose	[not]	z → t		X	
9. toad	[dot]	t → d d → t	X	X	
10. safe	[teɪp]	s → t f → p			X

◇◇

EXERCISE 26

Target	Child Form	Answer
1. tree	[fi]	coalescence
2. host	[hots]	metathesis
3. ask	[æks]	metathesis
4. behave	[hibeɪv]	metathesis
5. star	[tʃɑr]	coalescence
6. most	[mots]	metathesis
7. spoon	[fun]	coalescence
8. trick	[fɪk]	coalescence
9. tea cup	[kitʌp]	metathesis
10. spark	[fɑrk]	coalescence

EXERCISE 27

Target	Labial	Alveolar	Velar	Nasal
Ex: shoot		X		
1. limb	X			X
2. take			X	
3. farm				X
4. gate			X	
5. can		X		X
6. bake	X			
7. line				X
8. loop	X			
9. dog			X	
10. cheese		X		

EXERCISE 28 ◇◇◇

Target	Child Form	Sound Change	Labial	Alveolar	Velar	Nasal
Ex: *rope*	[wop]	r → w	X			
1. take	[keɪk]	t → k			x	
2. game	[meɪm]	g → m	x			
3. cone	[ton]	k → t		x		
4. coat	[kok]	t → k			x	
5. shoot	[tut]	ʃ → t		x		
6. win	[mɪn]	w → m				x
7. save	[feɪv]	s → f	x			
8. soap	[pop]	s → p	x			
9. loaf	[wof]	l → w	x			
10. goat	[dot]	g → d		x		
11. dog	[gɔg]	d → g			x	
12. thief	[fif]	θ → f	x			

◇◇

◇◇◇◇◇◇◇◇ **EXERCISE 29** ◇◇

Target	Child Form	Target	Child Form
1. Kay	[ke]	6. goat	[dot]
2. gate	[det]	7. go	[go]
3. sheet	[tit]	8. Joe	[dʒo]
4. Jane	[deɪn]	9. she	[ʃi]
5. kite	[taɪt]	10. Gay	[ge]

Sound changes:

t/k (5), d/g (2, 6), t/ʃ (3), d/dʒ(4)

Inconsistencies:

/k /   correct in *Kay*
        incorrect in *kite*

/g /   correct in *Gay, go*
        incorrect in *goat, gate*

/ʃ/   correct in *she*
        incorrect in *sheet*

/dʒ /   correct in *Joe*
        incorrect in *Jane*

Working hypothesis:

A comparison of the environments shows that there is a sound change only in words where there is an alveolar consonant. Further, the substitution is always an alveolar. This pattern suggests alveolar assimilation.

◇◇

EXERCISE 30 ◇◇

Target	Child Form	Target	Child Form
1. farm	[fɑrm]	7. dart	[dɑrt]
2. two	[tu]	8. back	[gæk]
3. took	[kʊk]	9. do	[du]
4. dog	[gɔg]	10. take	[kek]
5. dark	[gɑrk]	11. baby	[beɪbɪ]
6. tag	[kæg]	12. top	[tɔp]

Sound changes:

Initial word position: k/t (3, 6, 10), g/d (4, 5), g/b (8)

Inconsistencies:

/ t /   correct in *two, top*
         incorrect in *tag, take, took*

/d /   correct in *dart, do*
         incorrect in *dog, dark*

/b /   correct in *baby*
         incorrect in *back*

Working hypothesis:

Anterior stops are replaced by posterior stops (velars) when velar stops are in the word environment. This pattern suggests velar assimilation.

◇◇

Target	Child Form		Target	Child Form
1. shoot	[tut]		6. sheet	[tit]
2. case	[teɪt]		7. Jeep	[dip]
3. she	[ti]		8. goose	[dut]
4. go	[do]		9. Sue	[tu]
5. far	[fɑr]		10. suit	[tut]

Conclusion:

The sound changes are due to stopping and fronting.

Reasoning:

The sound changes occur without regard to context. For example, the /g/ changes in the word go, which has no final consonant, and in the word goose, which has a word-final /s/.

Target	Child Form		Target	Child Form
1. take	[keɪk]		5. toe	[to]
2. back	[gæk]		6. talk	[kɔk]
3. top	[tɑp]		7. shake	[kek]
4. bow	[bo]		8. sheet	[tit]

Conclusion:

Velar assimilation is occurring.

Reasoning:

The sound changes to velars occur only in environments in which there is a velar consonant.

EXERCISE 33 ⬦⬦⬦⬦⬦⬦⬦⬦⬦⬦⬦⬦⬦⬦⬦⬦⬦⬦⬦⬦⬦⬦⬦⬦⬦⬦⬦⬦⬦⬦⬦⬦⬦⬦⬦

Target	Child Form	Target	Child Form
1. thin	[tɪn]	6. thumb	[fʌm]
2. those	[doz]	7. the	[di]
3. them	[vɛm]	8. some	[fʌm]
4. sun	[sʌn]	9. see	[si]
5. safe	[feɪf]	10. same	[feɪm]

Conclusion:

The sound changes are due to labial assimilation.

Reasoning

In this sample, the sound changes to labials occur only when other labials are present. When labials are not present, the substitutions are not similar to labials.

EXERCISE 34 ⬦⬦⬦⬦⬦⬦⬦⬦⬦⬦⬦⬦⬦⬦⬦⬦⬦⬦⬦⬦⬦⬦⬦⬦⬦⬦⬦⬦⬦⬦⬦⬦⬦⬦⬦

Target	Child Form	Target	Child Form
1. cake	[teɪt]	6. goat	[dot]
2. shoe	[tu]	7. shoot	[tut]
3. go	[do]	8. key	[ti]
4. cheat	[tit]	9. Joe	[do]
5. show	[to]	10. Kay	[te]

Conclusion:

The sound changes are due to stopping.

Reasoning

The sound changes in this sample are not dependent upon phonetic context. Changes are made to stops even in the absence of stops in the environment.

EXERCISE 35

Target	Raised	Backed	Lowered
ɪ	o i̠ e	e o̠ i	o̠ i e̠
o	e ɛ u̠	u ɪ e	e ɛ̠ ɔ̠
e	ɪ æ u̠	ɔ̠ i ɪ	u ɪ ɛ
ʌ	u̠ æ ɑ	o̠ i e	ɪ æ̠ o
æ	ɑ e̠ u̠	ɪ e ʊ̠	NA
ɛ	ɪ æ o̠	ɪ æ u̠	ɔ ɪ ɑ̠
i	NA	e ɛ u̠	u ɔ̠ ɛ̠
u	NA	NA	ɪ æ o̠
ɔ	u̠ æ ɑ	NA	ɪ æ̠ u
ɚ	ɪ æ u̠	ɪ æ o̠	ɪ ʌ̠ ʊ

EXERCISE 36

Target	Complete	Tenseness	Height
Ci C<u>ɛ</u>	o ɪ i	ɛ e̠ ɑ	ɛ u̠ ɑ
Cɑ C<u>o</u>	e ɑ̠ æ	ʊ ɛ i̠	ɚ̠ ɪ u
Ce C<u>ɪ</u>	ɔ ɛ e̠	ɛ ʊ æ̠	u ɛ o̠
Cu C<u>ʊ</u>	ɔ ɪ u̠	ɛ ə o̠	e i̠ ɑ
Co C<u>ɪ</u>	o̠ æ i	ɛ e̠ ɑ	æ e̠ ɑ
Cæ C<u>ɪ</u>	e ɑ æ̠	o̠ ʊ ɛ	ɑ̠ u i
Cu C<u>ə</u>	a ə u̠	æ ɪ e̠	ɛ i æ̠
Cæ C<u>ɪ</u>	æ̠ ɪ u	ʊ ə̠ ɔ	ɛ e ɑ̠

EXERCISE 37 ◇◇

NOTE: For the dipthong exercises, you may have omitted the /e/ and /o/, which can be monophthongs or dipthongs. Some transcription practices use one symbol for both forms of the vowels.

Rounded	ɪ	e	o͡ʊ	ɑ	u̲
Tense	ɛ	o͡ʊ	u̲	ɪ	i
Diphthong	e	u	ɑ͡ʊ	æ	ɔ͡ɪ
Lax	u	e	ɪ̲	ɔ	i
Rounded	e	ʊ̲	ɔ̲	ʌ	æ
Tense	ʌ̲	ʊ	æ̲	e̲	o͡ʊ
Diphthong	ɛ̲r	ɑ	o͡ʊ	ɑ͡ɪ	i

◇◇◇◇◇◇◇◇◇◇ **MINI-QUIZ 2** ◇◇

DIRECTIONS: Match the letter of each term to the correct definition or example.

a. regressive
b. contiguous
c. alveolar assimilation
d. backing
e. labialization
f. coalescence
g. vowel raising
h. diphthongization
i. vowel backing

j. progressive
k. total
l. labial assimilation
m. velar assimilation
n. alveolarization
o. metathesis
p. monophthong
q. centralization
r. vowel lowering

1. __i__ process that might be occurring if /e/ is replaced by /o/
2. __a__ type of assimilation that occurs when the sound that changes occurs first
3. __m__ type of assimilation that has a sound change affected by /k/ or /g/
4. __e__ process that might be confused with labial assimilation
5. __r__ process that might be occurring if /ɪ/ is replaced by /æ /
6. __l__ EX: /sef/ becoming [fef]
7. __q__ process that might be occurring if /e/ is replaced by /ʌ/
8. __k__ type of assimilation that occurs when the changing sound and the influencing sound become exactly alike
9. __h__ EX: /ɑ/ becoming [ɑɪ]
10. __f__ EX: /spun/ becoming [fun]
11. __d__ process that might be confused with velar assimilation
12. __c__ EX: /kot/ changing to [tot]
13. __o__ EX: /wɪsk/ changing to [wɪks]
14. __b__ term used to describe a changing sound and an influencing sound side by side

◇◇

EXERCISE 38 ◇◇

NOTE: Obstruents have voiced and voiceless members; sonorants are only voiced. If a sound is voiceless or has a voiceless cognate, it is an obstruent.

Sound Pair	Cross Major Classes?	
1. /s/–/r/	<u>Yes</u>	No
2. /n/–/l/	Yes	<u>No</u>
3. /t/–/h/	Yes	<u>No</u>
4. /m/–/h/	<u>Yes</u>	No
5. /z/–/f/	Yes	<u>No</u>
6. /j/–/g/	<u>Yes</u>	No
7. /ʧ/–/d/	Yes	<u>No</u>
8. /v/–/g/	Yes	<u>No</u>
9. /θ/–/ŋ/	<u>Yes</u>	No
10. /ʒ/–/ð/	Yes	<u>No</u>
11. /ʃ/–/ʤ/	Yes	<u>No</u>
12. /j/–/ʤ/	<u>Yes</u>	No

◇◇

EXERCISE 39

Distinctive Feature	p	b	t	d	k	g	ʧ	ʤ	f	v	θ	ð	s	z	ʃ	ʒ
Sonorant	−	−	−	−	−	−	−	−	−	−	−	−	−	−	−	−
Obstruent	+	+	+	+	+	+	+	+	+	+	+	+	+	+	+	+
Continuant	−	−	−	−	−	−	−	−	+	+	+	+	+	+	+	+
Voice	−	+	−	+	−	+	−	+	−	+	−	+	−	+	−	+
Nasal	−	−	−	−	−	−	−	−	−	−	−	−	−	−	−	−
Strident	−	−	−	−	−	−	+	+	+	+	−	−	+	+	+	+
Labial	+	+	−	−	−	−	−	−	+	+	−	−	−	−	−	−
Coronal	−	−	+	+	−	−	+	+	−	−	+	+	+	+	+	+
Back	−	−	−	−	+	+	−	−	−	−	−	−	−	−	−	−

EXERCISE 40

Distinctive Feature	s	z	ʃ	ʒ	h	w	j	l	r	m	n	ŋ
Sonorant	−	−	−	−	−	+	+	+	+	+	+	+
Obstruent	+	+	+	+	+	−	−	−	−	−	−	−
Continuant	+	+	+	+	+	+	+	+	+	−	−	−
Voice	−	+	−	+	−	+	+	+	+	+	+	+
Nasal	−	−	−	−	−	−	−	−	−	+	+	+
Strident	+	+	+	+	−	−	−	−	−	−	−	−
Labial	−	−	−	−	−	+	−	−	+	+	−	−
Coronal	+	+	+	+	−	−	+	+	+	−	+	−
Back	−	−	−	−	−	+	−	−	−	−	−	+

EXERCISE 41

Sound Pair	Sonorant	Obstruent	Continuant	Voice	Nasal	Strident	Labial	Coronal	Back	#
EX: /s/-/m/	✓	✓	✓	✓	✓	✓	✓	✓		8
1. /ŋ/-/p/	✓	✓		✓	✓		✓		✓	6
2. /t/-/d/				✓						1
3. /g/-/f/			✓	✓		✓	✓		✓	5
4. /ʃ/-/h/						✓		✓		2
5. /θ/-/b/			✓	✓			✓	✓		4
6. /j/-/w/							✓	✓	✓	3
7. /ʒ/-/m/	✓	✓	✓		✓	✓	✓	✓		7
8. /ð/-/k/			✓	✓				✓	✓	4
9. /s/-/d/			✓	✓		✓				3
10. /n/-/r/			✓		✓		✓			3
11. /s/-/θ/						✓				1
12. /tʃ/-/ʃ/			✓							1

EXERCISE 42

NOTE: Child has difficulty with the [+ back], [+ strident], and [– coronal] features. The error with continuancy occurred only one time and would not be considered a problem.

Sound Pair	Sonorant	Obstruent	Continuant	Voice	Nasal	Strident	Labial	Coronal	Back
t /ʃ	– –		(– +)	– –	– –	(– +)	– –	+ +	– –
d /g	– –		– –	+ +	– –	– –	– –	(+ –)	(– +)
t /tʃ	– –		– –	– –	– –	(– +)	– –	+ +	– +
n /ŋ	– –	– –	– –	+ +	+ +	– –	– –	(+ –)	(– +)
t /k	– –		– –	– –	– –	– –	– –	+ –	(– +)

Bankson, N., & Bernthal, J. (1990). *Bankson–Bernthal Test of Phonology.* Chicago: Paradigm.

Bernhardt, B., & Stemberger, J. (2000). *Workbook in nonlinear phonology for clinical application.* Austin, TX: PRO-ED.

Bernthal, J., & Bankson, N. (1993). *Articulation and phonological disorders* (3rd ed.). Englewood Cliffs, NJ: Prentice Hall.

Chomsky, N., & Halle, M. (1968). *The sound pattern of English.* New York: Harper & Row.

Dawson, J., & Tattersall, P. (2001). Structured Photographic Articulation Test–II. Featuring Dudsberry. DeKalb, IL: Janelle Publications.

Dodd, B., Hua, Z., Crosbie, S., Holm, A., & Ozanne, A. (2006). Diagnostic Evaluation of Articulation and Phonology. San Antonio, TX: Harcourt Assessment, Inc.

Dyson, A., & Paden, E. (1983). Some phonological acquisition strategies used by two-year-olds. *Journal of Childhood Communication Disorders, 7,* 26–38.

Edwards, M. L., & Shriberg, L. D. (1983). *Phonology: Applications in communicative disorders.* San Diego, CA: College-Hill.

Gierut, J. (1989). Maximal opposition approach to phonological treatment. *Journal of Speech and Hearing Disorders, 54,* 9–19.

Gierut, J. (1990). Differential learning of phonological oppositions. *Journal of Speech and Hearing Research, 33,* 540–549.

Gierut, J. (1992). The conditions and course of clinically induced phonological change. *Journal of Speech and Hearing Research, 35,* 1049–1063.

Goldman, R., & Fristoe, M. (2000). Goldman-Fristoe Test of Articulation–Second Edition. Minneapolis, MN: Pearson.

Hodson, B. W. (2004). The Hodson Assessment of Phonological Patterns–Third Edition. Austin, TX: PRO-ED.

Hodson, B. W., & Paden, E. P. (1991). *Targeting intelligible speech.* Austin, TX: PRO-ED.

Ingram, D. (1982). The assessment of phonological disorders in children: The state of the art. In M. Crary (Ed.), *Phonological intervention: Concepts and procedures* (pp. 1–12). San Diego, CA: College-Hill.

Ingram, D. (1989). *Phonological disability in children.* New York: American Elsevier.

Jakobson, R., Fant, G., & Halle, M. (1952). *Preliminaries to speech analysis: The distinctive features and their correlates.* Cambridge, MA: MIT Press.

Khan, L. (1985). *Applications of phonological analysis: A programmed learning text.* San Diego, CA: College-Hill.

Khan, L., & Lewis, N. (2002). *Khan-Lewis Phonological Analysis–Second Edition.* Circle Pines, MN: American Guidance Service.

Lowe, R. (2000). *ALPHA Test of Phonology* (Rev. ed.). Mifflinville, PA: ALPHA Speech & Language Resources.

Mackay, I. (1987). *Phonetics: The science of speech production* (2nd ed.). San Diego, CA: College-Hill.

McReynolds, L., & Elbert, M. (1981). Criteria for phonological process analysis. *Journal of Speech and Hearing Disorders, 46,* 197–204.

Pollock, K. (1994). Assessment and remediation of vowel misarticulations. *Clinical Communication Disorders, 4,* 23–37.

Pollock, K., & Keiser, N. (1990). An examination of vowel errors in phonologically disordered children. *Clinical Linguistics and Phonetics, 4,* 161–178.

Secord, W., & Donohue, J. (2002). Clinical Assessment of Articulation and Phonology. Greenville, SC : Super Duper Publications.

Shriberg, L., & Kent, R. (1995). *Clinical phonetics.* Needham Heights, MA: Allyn & Bacon.

Smit, A., & Hand, L. (1997). *Smit–Hand Articulation and Phonology Evaluation.* Los Angeles: Western Psychological Services.

Stampe, D. (1973). *Dissertation on natural phonology.* Unpublished doctoral dissertation, University of Chicago.

Stoel-Gammon, C. (1990). Issues in phonological development and disorders. In J. Miller (Ed.), *Progress in research on child language disorders* (pp. 255–266). Austin, TX: PRO-ED.

Stoel-Gammon, C., & Dunn, C. (1985). *Normal and disordered phonology in children.* Austin, TX: PRO-ED.

Weiner, F. (1981). Treatment of phonological disability using the method of meaningful minimal contrast: Two case studies. *Journal of Speech and Hearing Disoders, 46,* 97–103.

Winitz, H. (1975). *From syllable to conversation.* Baltimore: University Park Press.